"*Slapped Awake* is a cl
formation in the cruc
see the step-by-step p
ophers tell us is the v
book close. Its truth, beauty and insights regarding how to achieve
a good life, told in both verse and prose, will guide you through
the process of becoming an authentic human being."

Mary K. Radpour, psychotherapist

"This exceptional story demonstrates the value of embracing cancer as a part of life, and in so doing, discovering new and transforming meanings to life itself."

Fr. Douglas Schwert, St. Mary's Sewanee
Sewanee, Tennessee

"I read *Slapped Awake* in one sitting. I am grateful for the privilege
of reading this courageous and remarkable memoir. I am reminded of Raymond Carver's *A New Path to the Waterfall*, Jean Bauby's
The Diving Bell and the Butterfly, and Reynolds Price's *A Whole New
Life*… By the end of the text, I felt that I knew the writer. I could
trust her. I sensed the honesty in each emotion. She presents no
easy fixes or false pieties...Works such as *Slapped Awake* reassure
me of our common humanity."

Clif Cleaveland, MD
Author of *Sacred Space* and *Healers and Heroes*

"I have been savoring Debbi Hampton's writing, even her personal health and family updates, for six years now. Her words never
fail to resonate with me and soothe my soul. *Slapped Awake* is no
exception, capturing every nuance of breast cancer in ways that
are so brilliantly moving. I think it should be required reading."

Sara Williams, nine-year breast cancer survivor
NIH Sister Study Recruitment Coordinator

"There aren't many manuscripts that capture me the way *Slapped
Awake* did. Debbi Hampton's writing style and willingness to look
at tough issues of living with metastatic breast cancer while growing a family made for compelling reading."

Kathy LaTour, Editor-at-Large
CURE magazine

Living with Breast Cancer:
A Journey in Poetry and Prose

Slapped Awake
Deborah Lang Hampton

Westview Publishing Co., Inc.

First edition February 2007

Printed in the United States of America on acid-free paper

ISBN 1-933912-30-8

Cover photography by Steve Hampton © 2007

Book typography and cover design by Steven Wyandt

Published by:

WESTVIEW BOOK PUBLISHING, INC.
PO Box 210183
Nashville, Tennessee 37221
www.westviewpublishing.com

To my children

– blood and borrowed –
Hollin, Laura, and Chris

To my grandchildren

who give me a reason to get up every day
and help me rediscover the world through their eyes

And to my husband, Steve,

my soulmate and best friend,
without whose love and faithful presence
I could not have walked a single step of this journey.

Acknowledgments

Any book is both the work of one solitary writer, sweating it out over a keyboard, and of a team of people who support, encourage, critique, and do whatever they can to help the writer realize her vision. In a book about a life-transforming illness, there is an even wider circle of people, who work to keep the writer strong and as well as possible. All these wonderful people have helped bring this book to life.

First, my thanks to my health care providers, from the beginning to now. I have received superb, compassionate, and collaborative care from my physicians: Darrell Johnson, B.W. Ruffner, Larry Schlabach, Phillip Burns, Laura Witherspoon, Frank Kimsey, Arthur vonWerssowetz, William Oellerich, David Wendt, Dabney James, Quincy Chu, Mari Lilly, and Ann Mashchak. It takes a village… Special thanks and warm hugs also go to the best nurses that this old nurse knows, the chemotherapy nurses at the Chattanooga Oncology and Hematology practice: Sarah, Michelle, Angela, Becki, Dorothy, Deborah, Leeann, Jennifer, Misty, and Lenes.

Thanks for cheering me on in my encounters with cancer and rooting for me in the intense cribbage games against my husband during chemo!

Elaine Hill has been my peer counselor and partner throughout the course of my illness, my untiring listening ear, and my model for breast cancer support and advocacy. Thanks to Elaine for helping me through Y-ME and for her continuing warm friendship and assistance in countless ways.

I have had some life-savers along the way. My "Bridges" family – April, Tom and Chuck – held me up and loved me anyway. I can never adequately thank Ginny Young and Janice Robbins, who cared enough to pull me back from drowning when I was going down for the third time. My gratitude also belongs to Susan Ewing, LCSW, who helped me learn how to save myself and then become myself. I appreciate Connie Robinson, LCSW, for ably facilitating, with Susan, the invaluable therapy group for women with advanced breast cancer. Finally, Gerre Schwert, LCSW, has brought me an understanding of the mind/body connection and given me tools to use that connection to strengthen me.

Friends have been my mainstay. Some of you have cooked and coordinated my life. My Baha'i community arose with tenderness and constancy, helping on every level, week after week, offering everything from prayers to Persian cuisine. Some friends have been a good sounding board and seen me through dark times. Many of you have cajoled and prodded me to use my writing and to see art as an act of worship, especially when offered in service to others. There are so many of you, but my deep appreciation goes especially to Dorothy Edwards, Betty Morris, Lois Osborne, Mary K. Radpour, Helen Smith, Kathy Daugherty, Sara Williams, and Diane Oakley Winter. Hugs and huge gratitude also to Kim and Julian MacQueen, who generously have given us emotional and physical retreats in beautiful settings when we needed escape, respite, and healing.

Honest critics are important to writers. Thanks to the following for eagle eyes, a good ear for language, and helpful feedback: Jim and Elaine Hill, Sara Williams, Gerre and Doug Schwert, Dorothy, Betty, Hollin and Steve. Dr. James Markert gave valuable feedback on the medical glossary, and I appreciate his time and support. Joyce Jackson has a special place in my heart and the history of this book, reading it first with her excellent sense of language and an author's eye and then painstakingly and skillfully editing the manuscript. Her professional assistance was invaluable. I also extend my appreciation to Clif Cleaveland and David Magee, who gave me generous advice, feedback, and seasoned expertise, and whose encouragement helped me bring this book to completion.

I would not even have begun to write this book without the insistence of several people. My sister survivors in the "On with Life" therapy group pushed me to use the poetry to help share the emotional experience of breast cancer with a wider audience.

My friend, Steven Wyandt, nagged me lovingly (and doggedly!), not giving me any room to abandon or delay this project. His belief in my ability to bring this book to print made the difference between pushing through or giving up. His excellent aesthetic sensibilities and graphic arts talents are also manifest in the book's design. Thanks, Steven, for the countless hours you gave me to make the idea for this book into a reality.

Finally, thanks to Roger White, who has already gone from here to There. Roger was an incredibly gifted poet whose support and long-distance mentoring emboldened me to call myself "writer" twenty-five years ago.

Deborah Lang Hampton

Foreword

Twelve years ago, I reluctantly was thrust into beginning an arduous journey, the course of which I couldn't know. What I thought might be a little detour in my busy life became my life. In order to integrate the impact of facing a life threatening disease, I did what I had always done to try to make sense of my life: write. In the early days of breast cancer, I wrote in a frenzy. It was the only foolproof way I knew to try to make some sense of what was happening to me. Over the 12 years that I have dealt with breast cancer, poetry has been my outlet, the place I go to crystallize the experience, the place I go to tell myself the truth.

As the body of poems grew, I began sharing them selectively with other survivors and friends. I was overwhelmed by their positive response and encouragement to "do something" with them. I had seen quite a few fine books on how women coped with the diagnosis and initial treatment of breast cancer, but I did not find much about how we live with having had the disease for the rest of our lives, nor what happens if the cancer recurs. In many types of cancer, there is a significant and growing population of survivors who are learning how to manage and live with cancer as a chronic disease. This is uncharted territory in everything from medical economics to psychological coping. As this new trend unfolds, the artist's voice will be as important as the analyst's.

Like any other art, poetry is highly individual, and those reading it have a highly individual response. People usually smile over a grimace when you say that you write poetry. I know that I sometimes do. It's such an intimate, personal process and finally, the poet largely defines what poetry is – and who's to say it's not poetry? For my tastes there's an awful lot of mediocre -- even trite and terrible -- stuff out there. I've also had the joy of reading some work of others who have been through breast cancer that made me wonder if they had been reading my journals. Their imagery and tone faithfully reflected my own experience, sometimes giving form to my feelings. I don't know what "makes a poem mean", to paraphrase John Ciardi, but I know when I hear a good one, one that makes my bones ring like chimes.

To me, poetry should hit you in the gut, even if it's something as seemingly mundane as how a bowl of apples looks on top of the piano. It's all about truthfulness. Like humor, a good poem should surprise you and take you to a place of looking that you hadn't found before, or was even dangerous to get to. Maybe it brings you up over a hill and knocks you to your knees by what it reveals on the other side. It doesn't have to be grand or profound or epic in length. A poem should go deep inside the eye, or the heart, or the hope, or the dark places. Sometimes it should give you words for your feelings, even when you had not yet fully felt them. I want my poems to be searing word-songs. I hope that you laugh or gasp or think about them later. Most of all, I hope that they give voice to my own truths and that, together – writer and reader – we find the common verities that connect us as humans.

At the beginning of each chapter, I have included excerpts from Rumi, a poet from the Middle East who lived 800 years ago. His work has sometimes been my voice, my conscience, and my guide. Across the centuries, he still speaks powerfully. The razor edges of his poems lacerate our hearts, cutting through our defenses, down to the core. I have provided a bibliography and references in the appendix so that you can go to the source and full text of these wonderful renderings created by Coleman Barks. He has taken the stiff, formal, literal translations of Rumi from the original lyrical, expressive Persian and breathed life and emotion into them to astonish us with their freshness and relevance.

As I gathered my poems together I realized that there was a story that went with them, so the poems are the scaffolding for the story. The story is not just about breast cancer. Extreme events change us. This story also encompasses what I learned about myself, how I changed, what choices I made, and who I became because I had to face losing my life. There are parts of this story that affected a wide circle of people. They have their own perspective and their own stories to tell. This is my story and mine alone. I have tried to tell it honestly, even though that wasn't always easy.

I had to embrace it all. Each chapter was part of bringing me to the life that I have now, this precious life I have now.

The Guest House

This being human is a guest house.
Every morning a new arrival.

A joy, a depression, a meanness,
some momentary awareness comes
as an unexpected visitor.

Welcome and entertain them all!
Even if they're a crowd of sorrows,
who violently sweep your house
empty of its furniture,
still, treat each guest honorably.
He may be clearing you out
for some new delight.

The dark thought, the shame, the malice,
meet them at the door laughing,
and invite them in.

Be grateful for whoever comes,
because each has been sent
as a guide from beyond.

- Rumi

Birds make great sky-circles
of their freedom.
How do they learn it?

They fall, and falling,
they're given wings.

- Rumi

Chapter 1

Coming out of the anesthesia, my mind was hijacked by scattered images of recent weeks. I could hear the music of the rivers in Costa Rica and smell the wood smoke of the Guaymi Indian settlement. I could see the corduroy wrinkles of the mountains below us, dotted with snow-capped volcanoes, as we flew home to Tennessee. I remembered my mental list of things to do when I got unpacked: register Hollin for school, buy Daddy a birthday present, make an appointment with my surgeon to check out a funny bump I found while on my trip.

I swam my way to the surface of consciousness, up through the cottony anesthetic currents to the fluorescent-lit summer day in the recovery area. My husband's face was over me as I tried to focus. "Where's Dr. Burns?" I asked.

"He checked on you several times, but you had trouble waking up. He had to go on to his next patient."

"What did they find?"

David's face was arranged carefully as he said the words

that changed my life forever, "It was cancer."

Weeks before, I was traveling in Costa Rica and got dysentery. I was as sick as I had ever been, reduced to helplessness after only an hour of dysentery. I didn't care about the people standing around me as I lay on the side of a red dirt road. Their faces showed an odd mixture of concern and embarrassment as my belly spasms drew me up, knees to chest. I was already so dehydrated, I wondered if I might die before we could drive the hour over river rocks and dirt road in a banged-up old Landrover, to the highway that would take us back to a southern town in Costa Rica, another four hours away. I didn't yet know it, but the red dirt road I was lying on would lead me not just back to town, but to my future.

I have spent a lot of time in Third-World countries. I am fanatical (probably to the point of obnoxiousness) about what I eat or drink, knowing that when you're going to be somewhere for just three weeks, days spent sick can take a significant bite out of a trip. I boil, filter and carry my own water. I only drink coffee or something hot that I know has been boiled. But among those in my traveling group, I was the only one who got dysentery. Maybe it was the re-warmed coffee drunk in the small Guaymi Indian settlement the afternoon before; maybe it was a Divine Hand reaching down and plucking me out of my old life.

I had brought my daughter Hollin and a friend's fourteen-year-old daughter to Costa Rica for three weeks. We were meeting up with old family friends who serve as itinerant teachers to indigenous people living on the border of Costa Rica and Panama, in the most glorious geography that could ever move your heart. Parviz, the husband in the family, traveled from their home in San Isidro del General to the mountains in the south to teach the Guaymi and Bribri people. Now desperately sick with the worst intestinal cramps I ever had, I rode back to San Isidro in Parviz's well-worn Landrover and I wondered, How could this have happened to me? I was so careful! Parviz had seated me on newspapers and plastic trash bags to spare the car's upholstery. Still in the grip of dysentery, I was not a pleasant traveling companion, and Hollin's eyes were wide with concern. I was nearly beyond caring, marveling that I could pass from upright and able to dehydrated and shocky in just an hour.

Back in San Isidro, at our friends' home, I took a shower, leaning shakily against the bathroom wall, the cold water washing me clean. I put on a fresh nightgown and sipped the tea that their son brought me. The Lomotil was finally working and they had gone for antibiotics.

I was lying in bed, limp. The fan blew gently on me, cooling the afternoon air in their house on the Pan American Highway. I rested my hands on my chest and closed my eyes. With my right hand over my breastbone, I felt something odd. I looked down and I saw it. Where the rib joins the breastbone, the right side was noticeably higher. I looked again and felt it carefully, exploring the edges at the border of my breast tissue, comparing it to my left side. It wasn't my rib. There was a lump, hard as a walnut. OhGodohGodohGodohGod. If I hadn't been so dehydrated, I might not have noticed this place for months. I knew with certitude that this was bad.

The date was July 1, 1994. I was 1000 miles and three weeks from home. I put the worry up on a mental shelf and finished the trip.

When I returned to Tennessee, I called my surgeon, a wonderful doctor who had specialized in breast disease and who had been following my lumpy, bumpy breasts for ten years. I saw him on August 1.

When he examined the area, I watched his face change. "Dr. Burns, you're no poker player," I teased him, hopefully.

He smiled thinly, with care and tenderness in his eyes. "I'm taking this out tomorrow," he said. "Carol will help you with scheduling and I'll see you in surgery in the morning."

I had hoped that this could be explained away by a professional. Now I was scared.

I had gotten mammograms since my mother was diagnosed with breast cancer 10 years before. I did breast self-examination regularly and had clinical breast exams once or twice a year. I had done all the right things and yet here we were. This inner-quadrant tumor, in this uncommon place, had not been pulled into a mammogram and was now just discernible against the background of ribs and breastbone.

Generally, I have a vivid memory, secured by all my senses, but August 2, 1994 is shot full of holes. I remember just threads of the day and the two weeks that followed. I went numbly to the OR for an open biopsy, basically a lumpectomy. Dr. Burns hoped that he could get the tumor out with clean margins, with no microscopic evidence at its edges of any more tumor. We were all hoping that the immediate pathology exam, a cell-thick "frozen section" looked at under a microscope while I was under anesthesia, would come back negative.

"It was cancer."

The words hung in the air. Every landmark that had defined "normal life" for me had just been obliterated.

A week later, Dr. Burns was taking the stitches out of my biopsy incision. We were about to have "the talk." My pathology report showed a two-centimeter tumor, invasive lobular breast cancer, one of the less common types of breast cancer, and the edges of the tissue still showed cancer. That meant that this stuff was still there in my chest. I sat up and we discussed what to do next. I was fairly small-breasted, and the doctor had taken a sizable divot in removing the tumor, about one third of my breast and some underlying chest muscle. There was no real cosmetic advantage to cutting the cancerous area more widely. The next logical step was a mastectomy. Only, nothing felt logical right now. Nothing made good sense. I knew in my head that the choice of a mastectomy was right. I was having a perfectly controlled and sane conversation with my doctor, but my mind was shrieking. My daughter had just turned 10. I was 42 years old. How could this be happening? All I could think was, Take the breast off as soon as you can. Get the cancer out of me! I want to live. I want so much to live. I want my life back. I just want my life back!

My mastectomy could not be scheduled for two weeks. The first weeks after my biopsy and diagnosis were bizarre. I could not sleep. I roamed my house at night, restless and preoccupied. The pure adrenaline of fear stoked my energy. This new and difficult reality constantly occupied my mind. I was flattened by the weight of my thoughts. The possibilities and worries droned on and on in my head, hour after hour. I would not know until after the mastectomy if the cancer had already spread to the lymph nodes under my arm. Would I need chemotherapy? Would I need radiation? Could I return to work? How sick would I be? How much function would I lose in my arm because of the mastectomy? What would I look like?

The real riptide under all of this was the unavoidable list of the most basic questions: What if the cancer was already in my lungs or liver? Am I strong enough to face this? Am I going to die? How much might I suffer? Who will raise my daughter?

I prayed and prayed and prayed, disconnected from the words I uttered but compulsively saying them. One morning, alone in the house, torn between terror and hope, I went downstairs to my garage, closed myself in, and literally screamed prayers.

The day of my mastectomy finally came up on the calendar. Dissociated thoroughly by that time from the level of fear that I had sustained for weeks, I only remember that the pre-op nurse who helped me was herself a cancer survivor. She had been through surgery and chemotherapy and there she was, taking care of me, then going home and taking care of her children, six years after her diagnosis. Six years! I hung onto that number.

I woke from my surgery, swaddled in a breast binder, a Hemovac surgical drain sticking out of my chest. I was surprised that the mastectomy site itself was painless. The only thing that really hurt was under my arm, where the surgeon had removed the lymph nodes. I couldn't raise my right arm at all, and it felt as though bands of strong elastic ran like a cord from my armpit to below my elbow. Since managed care was beginning to dictate hospital stays, I stayed in the hospital for a day. Before I left the hospital, I got the results of the report on the lymph nodes. They were clean, there was no evidence of cancer there! I felt able to breathe for the first time in weeks.

As I was getting dressed to leave, the doctor came in to change my dressing and I got my first look at myself without my right breast. For me, it wasn't a traumatic event. I was so relieved just to have the cancer out of me that the slim incision line was a welcome confirmation that we had taken care of the cancer.

For Dr. Burns

With sculptor's hands
you press the clay of me
back together
seamlessly.
Neither diminished nor disfigured
I feel distilled
Pared to my essence
streamlined

smoothed
sleek as a dolphin
flashing in the sun.

It took about a week for the full pathology report to be complete and available. At my upcoming appointment with Dr. Burns, we would review the full report, which would give us a fuller picture of how aggressive my breast cancer was. We would be talking about what, if anything, to do next. I wanted to be prepared for that discussion.

When I had my biopsy, I had gone to the bookstore the next day, thinking that I would get a book about breast cancer to bone up on the latest knowledge and treatment. I strolled into the Waldenbooks store and up to the shelf of women's health books. There was a big section on breast cancer. I was frozen in place. I couldn't even raise my hand to take a book from the shelf. I thought, I'm going to throw up. I stood for many minutes, mastering my nausea, blinking back tears, until I could take two titles from the shelf. I paid for them and hurried out of the store, to the refuge of my car. It took another three days before I could open the books and read them. It was just too much to take in at once. I could only stand so much truth at a time.

The human spirit and psyche are amazingly adaptable and resilient. Just three weeks later, I was ready to present a well-reasoned case for preventive mastectomy to my surgeon. I had done my homework and found that my kind of breast cancer had a higher chance of occurring in the other breast as well. My main concern was to stack the deck as much as I could to ensure that I would live to raise my daughter, Hollin. My second concern was to take as aggressive a treatment approach as I could so that if my cancer ever returned, I wouldn't be second-guessing myself and wishing that I had pursued all reasonable options.

At my doctor's appointment, we reviewed the full pathology report, which showed a middle-grade cancer, neither indolent nor raging. I talked about my desire for a prophylactic mastectomy. Dr. Burns asked that I postpone any decision about additional surgery until I was well-healed and had also seen a medical oncologist. I was willing to wait but kept the idea alive for myself. A medical oncologist could help us decide if I needed further treatment.

As the weeks moved into the autumn, I was increasingly aware that breast cancer was forcing upon me an unexpected education. One of the early lessons of cancer as my teacher was the crazy paradox of the disease as both the scariest thing that had ever happened to me and a blessing of being slapped fully awake. The keen awareness of the possibility of losing everything I knew heightened my senses and rattled my soul. I felt as though my "receivers" were all wide open, almost to the point of pain, exquisitely tuned and scanning, scanning.

In the Early Days of Cancer

These days a bogeyman lurks in every closet.
With each cough
> *each headache*
> *each skeletal twinge*
I wonder if metastatic tendrils
are insinuating their way into my vitals,
or are these turncoat cells
> *as smitten as my newly wakened soul*
by the softness of my child's cheek in sleep --
the sweetness of the stars?

I set up the appointment with the medical oncologist to talk about whether further treatment would be a benefit. The prospect of chemotherapy terrified me. I remember when I was first diagnosed, I thought, I don't want to die, but I really don't want chemo. My only knowledge of chemotherapy was archaic nursing practice from my former career and memories of people deathly sick and debilitated from vomiting. And for whatever perverse reason, anyone and everyone who had a chemo horror story wanted to share it with me. It also seemed that wherever I went, people were talking about cancer, with that distant but ardent fascination of spectators at a disaster.

Duet

(overheard)   *(to myself)*

"She left three
little children, you know…"

    O God –
    Give me healing and wholeness
    and belief in my wellness.

"Those last weeks
just wore her family out.
No one slept a wink."

    My doctor, my friend –
    Give me hope and honesty,
    kindness and your knowledge,
    and brotherly shoulders to lean on.

"I heard that even with
as much morphine
as they dared to give her,
she screamed and screamed."

    O God –
    Give me courage to fight
    with all my strength this interloper
    who has breached
    the walls of my life,
    and also to learn the lessons
    he would teach me.

"She was just a shell of herself   *Give me love for those few*
at the end. You wouldn't have even   *who are well-meaning,*
known her – just skin and bones."   *but ill-timed...*

"And now her husband   *...and patience with them any*
left with those children to raise –   *who simply stumble headlong*
Such a pity..."   *into my pain and fear.*

When I went to see the oncologist, I had a moment of leaden feet again, reluctant to cross under the awning that said "Cancer Center," as though that physical act would drive the spike of the truth of my cancer deeper into my center. The old familiar nausea came in a wave over me for a second, and then I walked in.

B.W. Ruffner was a kind and seasoned oncologist. I liked him immediately. He and I talked about systemic IV chemotherapy and my desire for a preventive mastectomy. He supported my wish to have the other breast removed, giving an interesting genetic pedigree for my remaining breast. He said I now had two "first degree" relatives who had experienced breast cancer: my mother and the breast I had already had removed for cancer.

We also discussed chemotherapy. It was not a standard treatment at that time for women whose lymph nodes were negative. He felt that I had about a 90% chance of remaining cancer-free for five years if we did nothing else. Dr. Ruffner explained that if we used a regimen of Cytoxan, methotrexate, and 5-FU in eight treatments over about six months, it could add another 2-3% to lessening my chances of recurrence. He was not, however, eager to press me in that direction. In fact, he made clear that there is no "free ride" with chemotherapy and that if I chose to pursue that course, he would be watching my side effects very closely.

Five years seemed to be the magic finishing line that was the basis for survival statistics. I wished I could look out beyond five years and have a sense of my chances of recurrence. Five years seemed so soon. Hollin would only be fifteen. She wouldn't even be out of high school. How could I not take the best chance I could get?

I talked to the doctor about my fears of chemotherapy. He was the third physician who told me the same thing: that in the past several years, the biggest advances in cancer therapy were in the area of very effective drugs that lessened and often eliminated the nausea and vomiting that had made most chemotherapy hell for cancer patients in the past.

I decided to opt for the chemotherapy. He said that he would send a report to Dr. Burns and, presuming that I would proceed with the other mastectomy, as soon as I healed, we could begin the chemo.

During these early days of adjusting the focus of my life on breast cancer, it was difficult to get used to my friends and co-workers treating me differently. Either people were cautious about talking about my illness, treating me as though I were fragile, or they identified me as some kind of icon or hero for bravery. This change left me often feeling alone and lonely. I love to connect with people through joking and teasing and that kind of interaction virtually disappeared. I guess that many people thought that this was just too serious a situation to make jokes. That changed dramatically one wet, Sunday morning.

Late, by myself, in the boat of myself,
no light and no land anywhere,
cloudcover thick. I try to stay
just above the surface, yet I'm already under
and living within the ocean.

- Rumi

Chapter 2

I sang for almost ten happy years in a five-piece band called "Bridges." We performed an eclectic blend of everything from rock to folk, from bluegrass to gospel, to a capella doo-wop and jazz. The friends in that band were truly my second family and had been wonderful throughout the two months since my diagnosis. A week or so before my second mastectomy, we were performing at a huge, local craft fair in Northwest Georgia, at Prater's Mill. The weather in mid-October is usually gorgeous, but that weekend, there was a deluge of Biblical proportions. Vendors and hardy souls were still there, and people slogged through the mud and puddles, soaked to the skin by the driving rain, yet still enjoying the beautiful hand-crafted items for sale and traditional Southern foods and music.

Our irrepressible band member, Steve Hampton, sidled up to the microphone about ten minutes before we were to start playing and announced across a vast field to all assembled there, "The wet tee-shirt contest will begin at 10:15." This got some good laughs, including from us. Then he got up again to the microphone and announced, "And Debbi Bley will be appearing in the abbreviated wet tee-shirt contest at 10:20!"

I got hysterical with laughter. It felt so good! I thought, with a gasp, He thinks I'm going to live! He wouldn't make a joke about me if he thought I was going to die. I had felt so isolated and this joke had connected me in an old, familiar, welcome way to my friends and to myself.

In late October, I had my simple mastectomy on the left. Seeing myself without any breasts at all for the first time was unexpectedly startling.

Breastless

Standing breastless
before the mirror for the first time
My right side transected by a slender pink crease
My left – a wound still encrusted with dark blood,
bruised yellow and purple –
The Hemovac emerging from my side
like some alien link to fuel or air…
I am blanketed in an eerie sensation:
the paradox of strangeness
and familiarity embracing.
My ontogeny seems indeterminate again:
Will I be fish or fowl?
I feel apart not only from my gender
but my species
with no landmarks that say "human"
across the empty topography of my chest.
And yet
as though I belong profoundly and fundamentally

to a larger world
A universe of beings
who might not be so easily dispatched –
  identified, categorized, pigeonholed –
But into whose souls
  one would have to peer
  to seek the true nucleus of "being."

  This was the beginning of a time of great introspection for me. If I didn't look like a woman any more, in fact, if my chest didn't look even human any more, how did I define my reality? What did I believe about it? How important was the physical part of me? What did it mean to be a woman? Even though I regard myself as very accepting of others, I became aware of how reflexively and subtly I tended to assess things based on physical appearance. Now I was on the receiving end of this and in a new position. When people who knew what I had been through for the past several months greeted me, their gaze unconsciously went to my chest first.

  As a member of the Baha'i Faith, I believe that my essence is my soul and that my body is a transient thing. I knew that in an abstract kind of way, but losing my breasts made me have to wrestle with that truth hand-to-hand. The threat of a possibly fatal illness focused me and challenged me more urgently to clarify that belief. The undercurrent of these questions would keep me stirred up for a long time and bear me along into unfamiliar territory.

  Several weeks after my second mastectomy, it was time to begin the chemotherapy. I was really scared. I didn't know how sick the medicines might make me. It seemed that each treatment decision required a deeper and more complete act of submission on my part. Used to having to take care of myself and feeling safest when I was in control of that, I was having to give myself over to trust in a whole new way, and it was hard for me.

I drove myself to Dr. Ruffner's office, not really knowing what to expect beyond the drug information sheets I had read as part of giving my consent to be treated. I had expected that getting chemo would involve a very clinical setting in a treatment room by myself. What I experienced that first day, and what I have experienced since, was very different from what I had expected.

First Day of Chemotherapy

In white wicker chairs with flowered cushions
    we sit, side by side
    as though on a cruise
    or at a garden party.
IV's hang above us and hold us tethered in plastic embrace.
I am a new inductee in this fraternity,
my first day of chemotherapy a rite of passage.
I watch the Cytoxan drip into the IV chamber
and see the methotrexate tint the tubing yellow
    before it disappears into me.
I call up images of scouring my interior landscape
    for any fugitive cells
    that might be hobo-ing their way to a new home
    in my liver or my bones.
I glance furtively at those next to me:
    How is his color?
    How much hair has she lost?
I am met by open smiles.
    We bare our souls to one another
    before we even exchange names.

"What kind of cancer do you have?"
We do not shy away from the word
            that once struck horror in our hearts,
but take grim comfort in naming it aloud –
            our common companion.
In this room
            there is no need for disguise or artifice.
            Midnight has long since struck
                        and we are unmasked.

I went home that afternoon and waited to see how I would feel. I had a little nausea the next day, and I discovered that the anti-nausea drug that the nurse had given me intravenously brought my lower GI tract to a screeching halt. Once I figured out how best to cope with that, I felt surprisingly well. This time began six months of weekly visits to the doctor's office, either for weekly blood work to monitor my white blood cell counts or to receive my treatment. Throughout the winter, my calendar and my cells' own clock settled into the routine of chemo. I arranged my life around doctors' appointments, the effects of treatments, and the up and down swing of my blood counts. It seemed that everything from how I structured my time to what was important was pressed relentlessly through the fine-screened filter of breast cancer.

During this time, I wondered how my daughter was really doing. She had asked me when I was first diagnosed in her blunt, forthright way, "Are you going to die?"

I answered her as honestly as I could. "I don't think so, Hollin. Breast cancer can be a serious disease, but we took the tumor out when the doctor took my breast off. Now I'm taking chemotherapy just to be as sure as we can that there are no more cancer cells. We're doing everything we possibly can to make sure that I get well and stay well."

I felt that Hollin had pulled inside herself. I didn't know if she was just satisfied with my answer or if she was suppressing the fear that I might die. Periodically, I would give her an opening to talk, but she wouldn't take it. Over the next months, however, her fear bubbled up unexpectedly, like when she suddenly asked, "What if you die before I'm eleven?" Once she related a dream to me about our going somewhere, the two of us. She had to drive the car, even though she didn't yet know how to. She was to be left somewhere and couldn't go where I was going.

One time she got very angry with me when I couldn't help her with her math homework. "I wish I had a different mother!" she yelled.

"Boy! You're really angry with me, aren't you?" I responded. "Is this about your being afraid that something will happen to me?"

She dissolved into tears, sobbing, "I'm afraid, I'm so scared." I held her and finally she said, right from her gut, "I wish I had a different mother so I didn't have to face the pain of losing you."

Her honesty and full embrace of her fear led to some wonderful discussions about all the "what ifs," but I felt so sad that we had to explore those things when she was still so young. I would catch her looking at me sometimes, and I could see that my illness had taken something from her, too.

Locket

I do not mourn
the loss of breasts,
of outward appearance.

Perhaps I now see why they're called
*   "secondary" sex characteristics:*
*   They are secondary*
*   to what I do mourn.*
I grieve the early loss of innocence
*   for my daughter.*
My apparent maternal immortality
*   and omnipotence*
Should have foundered
*   on the shores of her adolescence,*
Not been pickpocketed
*   from her heart's tender locket*
at ten years old.
Since cancer came to me
Some days she holds me
*   in a solemn slate-gray gaze*
*   that is old,*
*   old.*

I approached my breast cancer initially just as I had approached all of my life to that point: grit your teeth, get through it, put on a cheerful face and, with this new opportunity, be the poster child for brave survivorship. I found, however, that this disease – its threat, its magnitude, the way it shredded my life from the inside out – was bigger than anything I could control or shape, even with my experienced hands. I was haunted, hounded by the focused beam of breast cancer shining on my life, calling me to ask myself how I wanted to live the rest of my life. With the end of my chemotherapy and the aggressive part of my treatment plans ending in the late spring of 1995, these issues were gaining more heft and presence.

Confetti

Last day
        last day.
A pulse in me beats full and strong
        last day of chemotherapy.
Seconds tick as chemicals drip into me
        Last day,
                last day.
I watch the clock in this new office,
        different from when I started treatment months ago.
        I, too, am different from when I started.
I faced screaming terror
and made it to the other side.
Last day,
        last day.
The IV needle slips its mooring in my vein –
        Out! Done!
I look for confetti
        balloons
        some celebratory ritual.
The smiles of other patients
        are bouquets enough.
Last day,
        last day.
I whisper a prayer for them
        and for me
        Last day.

As I finished my treatments in late May of 1995, I found myself restless and drifting. The world of family and friends around me seemed glad that my phase of active treatment was over and everyone seemed eager for things to get back to normal. The problem was that there was a great disconnect between what everyone regarded as what had been "normal" and the cataclysmic changes I had gone through for ten months and still had yet to figure out. I felt like I was in a free-fall. All the structure of medical appointments and all the professional support that had propped me up for nearly a year had been pulled out from under me. How did I know that I was really all right now? Couldn't we just do some preventive chemo every few months, to hedge our bets? How would I know if the cancer came back? What would I do if it did?

I felt so "other" in the world, as though I didn't really fit anywhere any more. On one hand, I found myself impatient with people who made a big deal out of things that now seemed trivial to me. On the other hand, I felt angry at myself for having the presumption to measure those things on what I came to call "The Cancer Scale of Catastrophe." It was hardly fair to expect others to have the same frame of reference that I had thrust upon me. I wouldn't have wished it on them. I talked with other cancer patients to try to gain some insight into how they dealt with feeling different. I reflected often and affectionately on one particular conversation I had with my parents' neighbor during the winter. He summed up that difference so well.

Tom Bray was the father in the family who lived next door to my parents in Maryland. He had come through pancreatic cancer, amazingly, and was still around to talk about it several years later. He had been through a tremendous ordeal with chemotherapy and radiation, treatment that had ravaged his digestive system. He was finally coming back from it all, able to eat and to gain weight and regain strength. Tom was, to me, a man of quiet, deep spirituality. I was eager to talk to him when I went home to Maryland for Christmas, after my diagnosis. I asked him what he had learned from his cancer experience.

He was quiet for a moment then said, "Well, Debbi, I've learned that I love my God. I love my wife and I love my kids. Those are the most important things." Then, with a twinkle in his eye and a chuckle, he said, "But I'll confess that I get a little impatient now with people who pole-vault over mouse turds!"

Yes! That was exactly it!

It was both a benefit and a barrier to have a newly calibrated set of scales on which to weigh the relative importance of things. I found that I could shrug off a lot more than before I had breast cancer, but that it often widened the gulf I felt between others and myself. It wasn't that I was a better person or more illumined than those around me were. I just had come through a disaster that had changed me and was hard to explain, even to myself.

Despite having a loving circle of friends and family, I found it difficult to find people who were patient with my need to talk my illness through, over and over again. The support group and the friends that I made through the local affiliate of Y-ME National Breast Cancer Organization were a refuge. Being able to help other newly diagnosed women also felt somehow redemptive. I was searching for some way to find meaning in all that had happened in the span of a year.

Hollin seemed to shift to another place as my treatments ended, too, although she approached this time and transition indirectly, in a way that stung me to the heart.

Recitations over Orange Juice

My surgeries are done
       Breasts gone.
       Chemotherapy through.
Months since the initial shock of cancer
       tore our family from its homey soil
       and shook us by the roots,
My daughter had suddenly taken
       to reading me the obituaries over breakfast.
She leans across the comics with pillow-printed cheeks,
sips her orange juice, and scans the ages of the deceased.
Anyone under fifty
       is recited to me with solemnity –
       and a hopeful face,
Waiting to hear my reassurances once again.
I pay her in the paltry pennies of probabilities
Hoping that my embrace
       will help cover a debt of certitude
I can never fully redeem for her.

We search this world for the great untying
of what was wed to us with birth
and gets undone at dying.

- Rumi

Chapter 3

I am the oldest child in my family. I'm probably a textbook picture of the firstborn, the prototype for overachievement and an Olympic-grade competitor in being the "good girl." Slap on top of all that an alcoholic family and a father who prized success as an unerring measure of worth and by my mid-30's, I was an emotional train wreck just waiting to happen. I can testify from my own experience and from observing others that the "perfect" life and all the control that goes with being hyper-responsible and super-compliant takes a tremendous toll. It's just exhausting. By my late 30's, I found myself depressed and despairing. Even my journals from that time eerily portend something serious coming. In one entry in the late 1980's, I sensed something happening on some undetectable level but I didn't know what. I wrote, "I feel like I am dying by millimeters."

I was reliable, competent, and productive but there was little joy. My marriage was an emotional desert. David and I were living in the same house, but our paths rarely intersected meaningfully. The sad truth is they rarely intersected, period. He stayed up watching TV until 3:00 a.m. or buried himself in work. He took family vacations with us less and less often and worked well over 60 hours a week. For my part, I stayed overcommitted and busy with the work of our faith and my music. I'm sure that the outside world saw us as industrious and devoted people, but the marriage, which had its challenges from the beginning, was withered. We wore a deep groove in the path of avoidance. What might have begun as each of us dealing with hurt became habit. That time was so painful for me, and I'm sure that it was terribly lonely and unfulfilling for him, too.

Just before we married, I had actually gone home from nursing school one November weekend to break the engagement with David. I had realized that we were not a good match for one another in temperaments, energy, or expectations of a marriage. Instead of breaking the engagement, I chickened out and set a wedding date with him. David is, at his absolute core, a good man. I adored his family. I convinced myself that I was lucky to be engaged and that what we had would be enough for both of us. It was a cowardly way to start something as serious as a marriage.

Now I was nearly a year into my cancer diagnosis, having walked what I thought was going to be an impossible road. With my treatments over, the questions about what I wanted out of life rang insistently in my ears. I didn't know much, but I knew that I had to make some fundamental changes. I hadn't come through all that hell for nothing, just to drift back complacently into a life that was sucking me dry from the inside out.

I came from a family that was all about appearance and not much about truth. I became very proficient at erecting pretty facades to maintain the illusion of stability and perfection. Even my journals from my adolescent years don't mention my father's alcoholism, my mother's emotional unavailability, my brother's drug abuse, and my grandfather's molesting me. I couldn't even look at those things committed to paper in my own handwriting. Anyone outside of my family would have seen us as solid community members. No one knew what went on in that house after five o'clock, about three martinis into the evening. My dad was a cruel drunk, aiming his vitriol at my brother. My mother stared down at her plate during dinner, rarely challenging his abuse. I resolved to turn myself inside out not to be another possible target for Daddy's mean-spirited attacks, hating myself for not being able to help or protect my younger brother.

We all colluded and became masters in co-dependence. I became a shape-shifter. I could be whatever you needed me to be for you. I didn't even have a clue about my need or right to become my own self. I tried on role after role. Being pretty smart and sociable, I was good at it, but underneath was always the quiver of insecurity, feeling like a fraud. I felt so totally woven into the mesh of family fabric that had shaped my view of the world.

Scion Song

The secret tide rushes in
and warms the sinews,
shames and exalts my blood.
Scion song:
I yield to its call.
The undertow sweeps me
past buoys and wreckage
that bear my father's mark:
        his persistent cynicism
        his private sadness
        his public suffering.

He seems a stranger to himself after eighty years.
In this riptide
my own conversations with myself are
> *sporadic*
>> *strained*
>>> *severe and stern*
Stretched taut on a loom
wrought of silver and steel
> *frost-ridden*
> *metallic*
> *remote*
> *yet familiar as the scent of home.*
This genetic heritage of emotion
> *holds me hostage.*
The harder I strive to break free
> *the more snugly the strands bind me*
> *within the chain mail fabric of family.*
I meet the mirror each morning –
> *the face is my mother's*
> *but his eyes gaze back at me.*

Working through the changes in me from my breast cancer was really lonely work. David sincerely believed that I was going to be just fine. It left little room for the terror living beneath my skin and my urgent need to figure out how to live the 89 days between the scheduled visits to the doctor every three months. I wasn't very good at taking care of the frightened kid inside me or being kind to the one who had just had a very tough year. A friend from work even gently reminded me, "Debbi, don't be so hard on yourself. You've been living on the outskirts of Hiroshima for eight months."

My illness had forced me to accept the kindness and help of others and to begin to leave behind suspicion or fear that I would somehow be beholden by taking in the good things offered to me. I had been good at giving; now I had to learn to receive and to stay open. It was hard to give up trying to be so tough. In growing up and in my adult life, the only way to be safe had been to be tough and go it alone.

Library Book

I had a moment of epiphany today.
I borrowed a library book –
highly recommended by some literary buddies –
And opened its pages.
In beautiful, stark language
the story begins
as a daughter returns home
to nurse her terminally ill mother
Through the last days of cancer.
When, on page four, I reached the words "liver metastasis"
I closed the book.
Through gritted teeth, I fiercely told myself,
"I can do this. I can."
Two paragraphs later
I drew a deep breath to lessen my nausea
and suddenly felt opened wide.
Free.
I, who still cannot watch any movie about Viet Nam
thirty years since my first preadolescent love
perished in the jungle three days into his tour of duty,
Surely do not have to read about death from cancer

only ten months after my own diagnosis.
Whatever am I trying to prove to myself?
I am strong enough.
   I can choose what I wish to be weak about.
The book made a satisfying thud in the return chute
Thirty minutes after I had checked it out.

My music became more and more of a refuge. Our group was playing out regularly at a local restaurant during the summer and fall of 1995 and that was so much fun. I felt alive, creative, and true to myself when singing and working with the other musicians and friends. We also had opportunities to do music that summer for our faith and in interfaith settings.

During this time, Steve Hampton became a source of great support and friendship for me. He didn't give me room to sterilize my responses about how I was doing, dealing with all the events of the past year. Actually, I spent a good deal of time irritated with him about this, thinking, Dammit! I'm being as clear-headed as I can be about this!

That was the problem. I was staying in my head very effectively about my whole life. One day, in exasperation, he said, "Debbi, can't you just say that you're scared?" With that direct permission to be scared, I dissolved into tears for the first time since those weeks in early August when I was first facing my diagnosis.

Steve and I had always had a kind of stormy friendship. He was strong-willed, passionate, opinionated, energetic, creative, funny, outrageous, volatile and incredibly generous with time, resources, and emotions. I admired his talent, and his intensity both attracted and scared me. Aw, let's be honest! I've always been a sucker for a guy with a guitar. Two other powerful, platonic attractions I had in my adult life had been musicians. One of the men was also a poet (and a fine one) so he really had my attention and my heart from the get-go. Music was always a doorway to energy and emotion for me.

In my family, my father had the corner on the market for strong emotions (primarily anger). There was never much sharing of feelings as I was growing up. We didn't even name them. I cannot ever remember my mother saying "I'm sad" or "I'm angry" if she was upset and crying. She would say "I'm nervous" or "I'm tired." For me, being with people who could share their emotions or express them was powerfully attractive. Since music was such a primary love of mine, that aspect enhanced the draw even more.

I had known for years that Steve had deep feelings for me. In the late 1980's, he had once told me that he loved me. The next week, he came back to me and said that he didn't expect or want anything in having told me and that he would never speak of it again.

Truth

You say you love me.
I know it's simply so,
as sure as sunrise and seasons
proceed along the ecliptic -
light and shadow.
You held me intimately in your gaze
a May evening
with eyes so full that
for a moment
my breath caught, overwhelmed
at feeling loved completely.

29.

Once again I know that
> *feelings abide in a realm all their own*
> *and can live on without ever*
> *traversing the bridge to*
> *the Kingdom of Choosing.*

What is, is.
> *You called it "sane."*
> *Truth is like that.*

Now, nearly six years later, I found that collaborating with Steve, as part of our association in Bridges, doing meaningful, creative work in partnership, was so precious and true and real to me. As I contemplated my long list of things and people I could lose if this cancer returned, my thoughts turned more often and surprisingly to him.

We sang out of town in mid-June, the two of us taking a booking that the whole group could not make. In the imposed intimacy of a long car ride, we talked and talked. The music went particularly well that evening and we were singing for a good cause. Riding the crest of happiness from the evening, we drove back to Chattanooga in the early morning hours. I found myself pulled almost magnetically toward speaking more frankly and openly about my life and about how his support and friendship had been a refuge for me, especially in recent months.

Half-shell

The road stretches out
an asphalt river
straight, slipping over the horizon

Summer steam rising.
Overhead the stars
prick pinpoints in
the canopy of night.
Minutes stack on minutes
settle into silence.
Driving deep into darkness
The intimacy born of a long car ride
    frees my heart
    and my tongue.
I offer words
that fly
        free
         feathered
          full-throated
unable to be gathered up again
        out in the world with life of their own
Changing me
        changing us
Filling me with certitude
        and leaving me with ripples
         of insecurity lapping at my soul
Feelings an incandescent bubble on my breath
My heart on the half-shell.

...Everyone
chooses a suffering that will change
him or her to a well-baked loaf.

- Rumi

Chapter 4

I think that sometimes there are confluences of events or circumstances that claim us. When I was trying to make sense of how breast cancer had changed my life, I wasn't looking for love. I felt as though an undertow had grabbed me and was bearing me relentlessly to some new place, throwing me exhausted and shipwrecked on the shore of a new land that I never would have had the strength to swim to. I was pulled under and pounded by this high tide, and I was fighting to survive.

Finally out of treatment and reckoning with my life, I felt anxious and lost. I was scared that the cancer would come back. I didn't know where I fit in the world any more. I felt blown apart and opened to feeling, the lump of ice that had blocked my taking a full breath finally melted.

Steve was often my confidante and my lodestone. My feelings for him were so strong, and I knew that he was also struggling. We fought to navigate this change in the nature of our friendship. I found the pull of his support compelling. He seemed to read and understand me with no need for translation. It was the beginning of the most painful time of my life.

Telegram

Homeless
    a castaway
    flung up on the shore,
I am gasping for air
    out of that life-filled, oxygen-rich environment.
Brought up fast from the amber depths of your eyes
I've got the bends.
Maybe it's the pain
    that is the messenger,
    the Western Union boy
    who rings the bell
    and sings to me,
    "You're alive. Can't you feel it? You're alive."

I had always needed rules to feel safe. When I was little, I believed desperately that if I only knew enough, I could take care of myself. I actually got books from the library on game rules and etiquette. I wanted to know how to do things "the right way."

Stepping off my own moral pathway (and, in some moments, leaping off it...) left me as exposed and vulnerable as I've ever been. My actions went against my faith, how I was raised, and my conscience. My involvement with Steve exploded every past notion of who I thought I was, and probably who everyone else thought I was, too. Paradoxically, I also was given the gift of loving him with a complete love that I had never experienced before, and a capacity to love that was deepened and deepened through this time of excruciating pain.

This experience stripped me to the bones. It ultimately made me clarify and re-choose my values and beliefs, perhaps consciously and mindfully for the first time in my life. I will always regret the pain I know I caused. In trying to make some kind of peace with this over the years in order not to be paralyzed or consumed by guilt, I've come to believe that somehow I had to be broken by the experience -- and it broke me in half.

I had to reclaim myself through all the suffering that came with that time. It pushed me to growth and, I hope and believe, to a level of genuineness, humility, and finally kindliness beyond what I had before. I had to move beyond duty and perfectionism to embrace submission and compassion, to come to a real understanding that we are all wounded and fighting our own battles, every one of us. I had believed most of my adult life that I was not judgmental, but when I was walking through the napalm of facing my own failings, I realized that I had often been glib and casual in urging others just to buck up and get their lives together. Before it was my turn to step into the fire, I didn't have a clue about real spiritual testing.

As my involvement with Steve intensified, we both were in anguish. This love had no future.

Canyon

Some love is a river
  wide in its course,
    lapping lazily at sandy shores
    filling streambeds
Nearly still in shallows
    many avenues to the sea.

Not ours.
We are all rocks and rapids
*   foam and falls*
whitewater with nowhere to go.
Perhaps in keeping to this narrow channel
*   a wider way will open itself to us*
*   in this world*
*   or the next.*
We'll cut a canyon with this love.

I looked at those around us who mattered to me so much. I was torn apart by the polar opposite tensions that boiled inside me: need and joy on the one side, guilt and fear on the other. In Steve, I found someone who cared about my heart, my interior life, who loved me totally for who I was and accepted happily how I loved him. Neither my full feminine power nor my big personality threatened him or scared him off. I could be weak without fear that I would lose myself, and he could call me to be strong when I needed to be. But the relationship proceeded dishonestly, steeped in fear, and I knew that huge hurt was inevitable.

I left my marriage in March of 1996. At that time, the fact that Steve and I were involved had become known and we were trying actively to end the relationship. Steve's own marriage was falling apart and there was, of course, tremendous pain, sadness, and anger in his own family. It was just an awful time.

When I left my marriage to David, I never had any hope or intimation that there was a future with Steve. While my life at that point was really messy, I made my decisions about ending my marriage to David cleanly and independent of any expectations about Steve.

I can say with absolute honesty that for me, divorce was 100 times more painful and difficult than cancer has ever been. I also know that had it not been for my cancer, I would never have known that I had the strength to leave the marriage and live on my own. Breast cancer was the fuel that was burning the bridges of my life behind me.

Steve and I grappled with the pull of our feelings for well over a year after I started living on my own. While it doesn't mitigate the emotional havoc that was flooding us and those we cared about, I can say with truthfulness and certitude that we were never casual about a day of this time, nor any single choice that we made, minute to minute. Sometimes Steve was strong. Sometimes I was strong. Sometimes we just weren't.

Many times, I thought that it would be easier to die. I sometimes wished that my cancer would return. At one point, I had 30 Percodan counted out on my vanity. I vacillated between fear that the breast cancer would come back and a hope that it would, providing an out that would resolve things for me, for us, for everyone. It would surely be easier than the unsuccessful mustering of my will.

After Dr. Ruffner retired, Larry Schlabach became my new oncologist. He was really kind and very competent, but my oncology appointments were times of terror. The fact that I had two friends, Sam and Mary, who were dying of cancer, heightened my fear. What if I had magically called the cancer back to me? How could I prepare for all the losses I anticipated?

Appointment

As my oncology appointment approaches
cancer is like a sponge

soaking up more and more of my thinking.
Just beneath my skin is fear
alive and real
omnipresent
irrational but palpable.
The fear is a stallion ready to streak off into the night at full gallop
dragging me behind
face in the dirt
the reins wrapped around my wrists.
Do I hold on or do I let go?
Sam's spindle cell sarcoma
and Mary's fulminating Hodgkin's
are the Greek chorus in this play,
The voices in the distance that remind me
that life is about progressive loss, a loosening of the ties to this world.
The answer must be to let go.

Some dear friends at work saw that I was falling apart in chunks. I never would have imagined that I would be the object of an "intervention." One morning, two of my loving co-workers pulled me aside and told me that I was not functioning and they weren't willing to watch me go to pieces any longer. They laid it all out, saying that I couldn't try to be my own counselor, that what I was going through was bigger than what I could handle, and that they weren't going anywhere until I made an appointment with someone to get some help. If I wouldn't, they would and they would take me. Their love and concern and the counselor to whom they sent me saved my life and put me on a long road to healing.

Suffering that you bring on yourself is in a class all by itself. A lot of my pain during this time was because I couldn't line up my feelings, thinking, beliefs, and actions. I was standing in the full Arctic blast of having stepped outside the safety and haven of my own morality. What could ease the pain? How could I make this easier? I had information on housing and jobs in Atlanta. I fantasized about running away. A turning point came one morning.

One morning, I stopped in at a local church and I was able to be by myself in the sanctuary. The church was familiar and comfortable to me, having been a part of the school where I worked as admissions director. I prayed and prayed – for guidance, for forgiveness, for relief, for wholeness and, yes, for some halfway solution and an easy way out. At one point, I was face down, lying full-length on the floor, mowed down by my own life. I came to the bottom-line issue for me: to whose Authority was I going to submit myself?

An actual warmth suffused me from head to toe. I knew that a Power higher than myself and a Will larger than my own willfulness was present, loving, and in charge. Knowing that truth in every cell of my broken body meant that I had to get my life lined back up with that Power. It was inescapable. I needed to be living my life integrated and whole, not shattered. It was going to be a long and difficult journey back but I was choosing it willingly and knowingly.

Chalice

There is purity in blunders made
　　with lowly, loving heart
　　that cannot be contained in acts of brittle piety,
　　duty-driven.
I know all about those acts of obligation, joyless
and dry as ashes.
Somehow, my heart unfolds.

I feel opened up inside
as I begin to embrace my weakness
and mistakes
> *and rinse them in the honest water of humility*
> *and good intent, and the plea for forgiveness.*

It seems that if love is the simple chalice
> *in which I bear my self to offer to you,*

Even if I stumble
and the cup is broken
> *and I lie spilled in the dust,*
> *that gift would be more acceptable*
> *than an empty, ostentatious cup*
> *and my heart locked away in fear and never truly offered.*

I begin to understand the powerlessness and poverty
> *about which I pray*
> *and to accept them as part of me.*

They are not something to fight against
> *or to be shamed by,*
> *but are gifts that define my place in the world*
> *and my need for love and mercy.*

A night full of talking that hurts,
my worst held-back secrets. Everything
has to do with loving and not loving.
This night will pass.
Then we have work to do.

- Rumi

Chapter 5

The summer of 1997 was full of great change. My divorce was final. Steve's marriage had also ended. We began a real relationship, cautiously but openly, for the first time. It wasn't easy. We had our children to consider. They were all still so raw. We had issues between ourselves that had laid dormant, issues that it would not have been appropriate to address before that time. There were residual feelings for both of us to deal with – good and bad -- and hopes and expectations to explore. Even being able to think about the immediate future felt strange.

As a single woman, my economic situation was precarious. I had been reluctantly trying on the idea of looking for another job. My position at St. Nicholas School doing admissions and financial aid had been the perfect job, but I simply needed a larger salary to meet my expenses. I had been active in Y-ME, the breast cancer organization that had provided a lifeline for me since my diagnosis.

In a recent strategic plan, Y-ME of Chattanooga had set a goal to have a paid staff member to coordinate its services. The

Board wanted to fill this half-time position by the early summer of 1997. I was on the Board's search committee, and we were eagerly anticipating hiring someone to help lead the day-to-day operations. In one of our committee meetings, President Elaine Hill came with some exciting news: a local hospital had offered to pay for the position and felt that it should be a full-time position.

I felt an electric shock of excitement and possibility shoot through me. I pushed my chair back from the table and said, "I need to resign from this committee. I want to apply for the position and I don't want any conflict of interest. I don't want to be privy to any more information that might give me an unfair advantage as you define the role and job description of a full-time Executive Director."

The organization went through an extensive search and interview process. To my delight, around the first of June, I got the call offering me the job of Executive Director. I accepted and began on July 1. I spent my next several years working every day trying to ensure that women facing breast cancer had someone who had been there to talk to.

Since the completion of my chemo two years before, I was taking Tamoxifen, the estrogen blocker that was the standard treatment for five years in women with estrogen sensitive tumors. A change in health insurance with my new Y-ME job had required a change in oncologists and I was getting to know my new doctor, Darrell Johnson. I felt well and my personal life was chugging along, finally with restoration of balance as the priority. During this time, I began to contemplate something that had never been important to me before: breast reconstruction.

I had never really mourned the loss of my breasts when I had my mastectomies three years before. My main concern had been to eradicate the cancer any way I could. After my mastectomies, I had managed the silicone breast prostheses and the pocketed, heavy bras that held them in place. I had purchased a special swimsuit in which the prostheses fit. I felt pretty good in my clothes, although I was careful about bending over if I had a vee-necked top on, since the bra and prostheses fell away from my chest at that angle. That was a little alarming to folks. I had never given a lot of thought to the ways my breasts had served me. My breasts had been a pretty part of my physical appearance and they had also nourished Hollin. I missed them. I was also in a time during which I embraced myself as a woman more fully than I ever had before.

Bouquet

Today I wished for breasts
for the impossibility
of ever offering them to you
as I once was
suede-petaled
tea rose bouquets.

I had to go to a formal event at the hospital early in the fall to mark the opening of a newly constructed area. I hadn't worn a formal dress since high school and looked forward to shopping for something pretty. I went to a local mall, to a store that had hundreds of formals of every style and color.

I tried on at least 60 dresses and nothing fit well or looked good. It was a hard day. I pulled on dress after dress and tried to stuff my two prostheses into the bodice, or put the bra back on and attempted to tuck and conceal bra straps. I felt so frustrated and sad. I got an achy lump in my throat and blinked back tears as the pile of unsuitable dresses grew. Finally, I just sat down in the dressing room and bawled and bawled. I was crying not only out of frustration but finally for the amputation of that part of me that made me look like any other normal woman. I eventually found a dress with a lacy overlay that held the bodice in place and purchased that. It wasn't my first choice of style but it worked.

Steve and I went to the formal (and I did look pretty darned good). We actually managed to laugh as I asked him to check on me after every dance or two to be sure that my tucked in bra and prostheses weren't going south toward my waist from gravity and the lack of straps to hold everything in place. Twice, I slipped away to the Ladies Room to rearrange all my gear. The notion of reconstruction was taking root firmly in my mind.

At our Y-ME support group, several of our members had completed reconstruction of various kinds. One woman had a TRAM flap reconstruction in which the surgeon uses abdominal tissue and muscle to create a soft, natural breast. You get a tummy tuck as a bonus, but it's tough surgery. Another young woman, Linda, who was very slender and an athlete, had bilateral reconstruction with breast implants.

I looked at the results of several kinds of reconstruction women had within my support group. Because I have had back problems, I wasn't eager to consider a TRAM flap, since using one of the abdominal muscles can affect support of the back. I looked at Linda's bilateral reconstruction with implants, however, with growing interest. She had such a beautiful cosmetic result. She had been frank and open with me in several meetings as I questioned her about the process of the surgery and period of tissue expansion over a few months post-op, as well as the nipple reconstruction. I kept trying on the idea and became more and more open to it, but kept my thoughts to myself.

At Thanksgiving, Steve and I became engaged and began planning for a wedding for February of 1998. It was a busy, happy time. He proposed to my daughter before he proposed formally to me, and we tried to include her in all the planning and house hunting. I put my thoughts about reconstruction on the back burner. We married on a lovely, February Sunday, in a ceremony full of music and poetry and the participation of our children and friends.

About two months after we had married, I made a visit to my surgeon, Dr. Burns, to talk about reconstruction. I was a little sheepish, actually. When he had performed the preventive mastectomy, I had noticed that he had left some extra tissue. I had asked him why and he told me that if I ever wanted reconstruction, it would give the plastic surgeon more to work with. I had adamantly said that I would never want reconstruction, that it simply was not important to me at all. Now, here I was sitting in a paper gown, waiting for him to come in so that I could ask him questions about reconstruction.

I asked him what if my cancer came back, how would we know, if there was an implant in place? He fixed me with a level gaze and said, "You're nearly four years out from your initial diagnosis. Let's be honest. Looking at the odds, if you were to have a recurrence, it would likely be in a distant site, like bone or liver metastases. The good news is that you're four years out and doing fine. If you want reconstruction, there's no medical reason not to do it." I made an appointment with a plastic surgeon, Dr. von Werssowetz (affectionately known as "Dr. Von"), for a consultation.

I knew that Steve would have been surprised to know that I was even thinking about reconstruction. He never had seen me any other way than without breasts. He was always tender and completely accepting of how I was, one time bringing me to tears by saying, "Your scars look like silk." He thought that I was complete as I was and once said, "I'm not overlooking anything. You are beautiful."

When I told Steve what I was thinking, he was flabbergasted. "I hope that you're not doing this for me in any way," he said, his voice full of concern. "This is not important to me at all. I've only ever known you as you are and you're beautiful just as you are."

All that I had been thinking about reconstruction over the past few months crystallized in my mind and I spoke, "I want to do this for me. This is a way of stepping beyond my breast cancer. I want to be able to shop for regular clothes like an ordinary woman. I want to buy sundresses and bathing suits and pretty lingerie that doesn't look like armor. But mostly, I see this as a way of moving another step past my cancer."

I told Steve that if I went ahead with this, these reconstructed breasts would be purely ornamental and that the skin on my chest would be even more numb than it already was, since it would have been cut more extensively. I said to him, "We need to be realistic about the results. The new breasts should look pretty good, but they won't be real."

In a moment for which I will always love him, Steve tapped his beautiful white dentures and, with a twinkle in his eye, said, "These aren't real either."

"I love your smile!" I said.

He grinned and spread his hands. "I rest my case," he said.

Over the next few weeks, I really pondered whether to proceed with scheduling the reconstruction. This was a big step and, while not as complicated as a TRAM-flap procedure, was still big enough surgery. Steve was careful to remain neutral and detached during that time, leaving the decision completely in my court, respectful of my right to decide alone. He did slip one night, around the time that I had decided to go on and do it.

"So, are we getting breasts?" he asked.

"Ha!" I crowed. "You said 'we'! Gotcha!"

It's a drum and arms waving.
It's a bonfire at midnight on the top edge of a hill,
This meeting again with you.

- Rumi

Chapter 6

I scheduled the surgery for early July. I went into the surgery with the idea that it would be a piece of cake and that I'd probably be back at work in three or four days. The plastic surgeon and I had talked about my desire for him to create a mammary fold, if possible, that would look natural below the new breasts, once they settled in. I reminded him that I was 46 years old and a little droop eventually would look good. He agreed. With implants, I was going to get a kind of perpetual firmness anyway. I could just see myself as a 75-year-old woman, with my saggy buttocks banging against the backs of my knees but firm breasts defiantly high and youthful on my chest. If there was a little realistic adaptation that could be made for age, that would be great.

In reconstruction with implants, the process is not unlike how a woman's abdomen expands gradually during pregnancy; the body does well with accommodating the need for the skin to stretch. After my surgery, every several weeks the doctor would inject more saline solution into tissue expanders placed during the surgery, until I was actually in an over-expanded state, bigger than the final size of 36C that we had agreed upon. This time of overexpansion would contribute to creating a loose soft pocket for the permanent implants. At that point, we'd just sit tight for some weeks as the tissue stretched and softened. My friend Linda had warned me, "During that time, your boobs will be so big they'll need their own zip code!"

The morning came for the surgery. Steve stayed with me in the pre-op area, and Hollin was ready to keep me company and help me post-op. I dove down into the amnesiac haze of Versed, knowing that when I awoke this time, when I reached for the bandage there would be breast mounds instead of empty flat terrain.

The recovery room team was rolling my bed back into my hospital room when I first remember waking up. Steve and Hollin were at the doorway, reaching out to me gently. My chest felt like the skin was going to split and I thought, I didn't think this was going to hurt very much! I looked down at the chest dressing and could see two little hills, round and firm. It was a welcome sight.

My plastic surgeon had immediately filled the expanders with 300 cc of saline solution, and the force of that was pushing against my tightly sutured chest muscles and skin. He anticipated that this would cause not only pain but muscle spasms, and it did. I could move my arms and hands in a very limited plane, able only to bend my arms from the elbow about 45 degrees before setting off a tsunami of muscle spasm that rendered me helpless and in tears. I couldn't reach my mouth or my bottom so I was totally dependent for all of my most basic needs. Generally tough about pain, I was a big baby. The night I spent in the hospital, the nurses got me up and I thought I was going to faint from the pain.

A little after midnight, rather than getting up or having to raise myself up, I actually wet the bed. I told Hollin through my tears, "I just peed the bed. Don't tell them. They'll make me get up!" She laughed and I cried some more. My night nurse turned out to be a big, muscular guy who was able to sweep me out of the bed in one smooth move without much strain on my chest.

The next morning, as my 23 hours allowed by insurance ended, I was sent home.

If this hadn't been summer, I don't know how I would have managed. Since Hollin was out of school for summer vacation, she was home and could help me. She was a great nurse. Steve's own portrait photography business provided the flexibility for him to come home between appointments to do the heavy lifting and check in on me, too. They both assure me that they propped me up on the couch in front of the VCR, popping in movies I had wanted to see for a long time, jostling me every once in a while to try to bring me around. I remember none of it. I was in a drooling, narcotic haze for five days.

Steve got in and out of the shower with me, since I couldn't reach anything to wash myself. Hollin wiped my bottom and spoon-fed me my meals. This was a lesson in total submission and it wasn't easy. I became aware on a whole new level what a control freak I am. I had to give that up completely.

After about five or six days, I started feeling better. I began to be able to move my arms in a more normal range of motion without pain dropping me to my knees. I got a good look at these new breasts and saw where we were headed with this process. The initial effect was of two half cantaloupes that sat high and round, nearly up under my collarbones, but I knew that they would settle in and progressively look more natural.

I felt a strange developmental kinship with Hollin who, at thirteen, was also getting breasts. My reconstruction reminded me of my own adolescence.

Reconstruction

This process strangely parallels
my adolescent daughter's development.
We sheepishly compare
her pubescent, budding breasts
to my own expanding, nipple-less Barbie boobs
and hug like interlocking puzzle pieces.

I felt like an adolescent again myself, excited about the growth of these new breasts. I had been an eager preadolescent, longing for breast development and my period, measuring my chest often to see if anything was happening, and even one time making myself a bra. I was about 10 years old and still flat as an ironing board, with not even the first little rosebud promise of breasts. In what must have been some of the first "image" advertising, I remember that Maidenform® Bras was running magazine ads with beautiful women dressed in diaphanous things and Maidenform® lingerie, gliding through exotic places, with the caption "I dreamed I (fill in the blank) in my Maidenform® bra."

I hand-sewed my dinky little bra from scraps found in the seat of Mama's sewing chair. I even included a little violet flowered inset and a red ribbon. Straps were lengths of 3/8 inch elastic. Oh, it was a beauty! I modeled it for Mama and Daddy and my dad proclaimed, "I dreamed I stubbed my toe in my Beanform bra!" I recall the moment as loving and supportive of my interest in all the things that were going to turn me into a woman. Some of that familiar feeling accompanied this new journey for me, too.

Reunion

This rebuilding is a restoration
on the barren site of my chest
where I've been razed to the bones.
The implants stretch my skin and muscle
as I birth these new breasts,
the post-op pain a kind of labor –
my plastic surgeon midwifing me along,
week by week.
These bogus breasts are facsimile –
Ornamental, I know –
but emblematic for me.
Four years after my mastectomies
I have chosen to step beyond my cancer.
One hot July evening,
I rummage through my bureau
and find the single silky slip with fitted bodice
that I crammed in the corner of the drawer
when I discarded stacks of alluring lingerie
years ago,
trading it all for flat front options.
I shake the wrinkles from its satiny surface
raise my arms
and slide it on.
It slips into place,
holding these saline-filled potential breasts
like a lover's hands.
I am suddenly weeping
not for loss,

but for a joyous finding,
An unexpected encounter with a long-lost girlfriend.
Stunned by the sweet, sweet strength of my own sexiness,
I revel in this reunion with myself.

After I returned to work, one lunch hour I went back to the store that specialized in formals, where the seeds of the idea of reconstruction had first germinated. I found a dress more daring in design and cut than I had ever thought to consider. It was a beautiful red dress, fitted and floor-length, with a low-cut fitted bodice and a slit to mid-thigh. It was stunning. I couldn't imagine where I would ever wear it (or if I would ever have the nerve), but I bought it.

That night I made Steve wait in the living room while I put it on. I didn't tell him what I was making him wait for, just that I wanted to show him something. I came down the living room steps and told him to open his eyes. "Sheeeee-it!" was his immediate response. I laughed and clapped my hands in delight. "That's the reaction I wanted!"

As the tissue expansion moved forward quickly, September found me at the promised stage of over-expansion and waiting to schedule the final surgery to put in the permanent implants. I had a funny thing happen one afternoon as I was walking from my office across the busy street to the hospital lot where my car was parked. It was a cool enough day that I was wearing a short-sleeved sweater and slacks. As I got ready to cross the street, a carload of young men drove by. The car slowed and one of the guys hung his head out the window. With the catcalling of his buddies as the background music, he hollered, "Hey, baby! You've sure got some big tits!"

It was the funniest thing that could have happened. I wanted to run after the car and tell them, "You don't even know the half of it!" I couldn't call up even a shred of righteous indignation from what should have been the affronted feminist side of me. I just sat down on the curb and laughed until the tears rolled down my face.

Finally, the day came to go back into surgery for my permanent implants and the nipple reconstruction. This time when I woke up from surgery, there was very little pain. Already, the completed breasts had mobility and settled lower on my chest, more softly and naturally. The nipple reconstruction looked great. When I finally had healed enough and had the go-ahead from Dr. Von, Hollin and I went lingerie shopping. It took a little looking and trying on to find brands that accommodated my roundness, but it felt wonderful to buy pretty things and matching things. Such a simple pleasure!

Looking back on the pain of the surgery and having to subject myself to the whole process that was involved in completing the reconstruction, I know that it was an important thing for me to do at that time. Every time that I had stood in front of the mirror each night, taking my Tamoxifen and seeing myself breastless in the mirror, I had the constant reminder of breast cancer. Reconstruction was a way to say to myself that I was well enough to move on. Given all the factors I considered at the time, I would do it all over again. It was a big part of my overall healing, and I felt whole again in a new way.

The morning wind spreads its fresh smell.
We must get up and take that in,
that wind that lets us live.
Breathe before it's gone.

- Rumi

Chapter 7

The several years that I was the Executive Director of Y-ME were busy, satisfying, and sometimes emotionally challenging. We were building a core of trained peer counselors to work with newly diagnosed women and women with recurrence, but the implementation of that system was not yet fully in place. The plain truth is that since I was the person in the Y-ME office, I was the most accessible when women were facing a crisis. I saw them when they were raw with the disbelief and terror of a new diagnosis or devastated by news of a recurrence. Sometimes they came to my door literally within minutes of leaving the doctor's offices down the hall. Y-ME was providing a vital service. It was a gift to meet so many women who were being transformed by their experience. I was their witness, watching them rise to heights of courage and fortitude they might not have known they had the capacity to attain. Some of the most exalted experiences of my personal as well as my professional life were through the women I met.

Sister Survivors

These women
> *These strong women*
>> *tested*
>>> *battle-scarred*
> *emerge from the crucible*
> *of their common ordeal*
>> *burnished*
>>> *great-hearted*
>>>> *golden*

These fine, strong women.

    The discouraging part, however, was that over and over the increasing prevalence of breast cancer, its random and renegade nature, and the tremendous cost, both emotional and material, to patients and their families were manifest every single day.

    It was hard for me (and new to me at that point) to become close to someone a lot like me, by virtue of age or circumstance, and then to lose her to death. So many names and faces go through my mind. There were mothers of young children, a feisty grandmother who used to go without a wig and proudly wear the Chiquita® Banana stickers her grandson had placed on her bald head, a formerly healthy runner in her thirties who married during her chemotherapy in full bridal regalia, pale and frail from treatment but still radiant. There was one woman with an aggressive form of breast cancer that rapidly recurred after treatment, who called me from the hospital crying, "Debbi, the cancer's taken my brain!" There was another woman who wanted to live long enough to be at her son's wedding, but who feared that her husband would see her as "fat" since the chemotherapy and steroids keeping her alive had put weight on her and she needed to buy a new "mother-of-the-groom" dress in a bigger size. There were the ones who weren't "supposed" to get the disease back but who did and who, passing my office after leaving their oncology appointment, broke down sobbing in my arms, their worst fear realized.

I kept my conversations with these women confidential, of course. If I took a call at home, I particularly tried to ensure that I had total privacy, but Steve and Hollin could infer that I was talking to someone who was hurting or scared, or that the phone call had delivered bad news to me. One evening Steve said, "Sometimes this is like knowing that you're going to die in a car wreck and every few weeks being forced to watch a movie in which someone dies in a car wreck."

Ah, the cascading effects of breast cancer. It bled all over me and those around me.

With early detection and the cancer confined to the breast, most women – about 95% -- are still cancer-free after five years. My view of the disease was through the telescope that homed in on women at the time of diagnosis or dealing with metastases. Some days, fanning the fires of hope – for myself and for them -- was hard work. Although I reminded myself consciously and often that the vast majority of breast cancer patients do fine, my emotional experience of the disease was rooted in the crisis points of breast cancer: diagnosis and recurrence.

Late in the spring of 1999, a wonderful avenue opened itself to me and gave me new reasons to be hopeful. Through my work with Y-ME, I was invited to serve as a consumer reviewer of breast cancer research proposals funded by Congressionally-directed money. This program started in 1992 through the fierce and effective lobbying efforts of the National Breast Cancer Coalition (NBCC) and breast cancer survivors. Survivors demanded more research money and built a convincing case for funding beyond what Congress appropriated to the National Cancer Institute. Today, this program is second only to the National Cancer Institute in its funding of breast cancer research. It is the second largest freestanding breast cancer research program in the world.

In 1993, the Department of Defense (DoD) was called upon to manage the program through its U. S. Army Medical Research and Materiel Command. While this marriage of breast cancer research and breast cancer advocates with the U.S. Army may seem strange, the Army has a long history of biomedical research in diseases and other health and medical problems faced by soldiers, not to mention that they have the structure and experience to run a big operation. Who would be better equipped to conduct a "war" on breast cancer?

In 1993, the NBCC asked that breast cancer survivors have a voice at the table where decisions were to be made about the research proposals, an inherently competitive process. That year, consumers served on the Integration Panel, the final decision-making board that selects the proposals to receive funding. It was soon apparent that having people who had actually experienced breast cancer was extremely valuable. In 1995, consumers also began serving on the Scientific Peer Review Panels, which review all proposals and score them so that the Integration Panel can then do its work. Interestingly, this model of consumer participation has become the rule for the core cancer research programs administered by the U.S. Army Medical Research and Materiel Command and has been emulated by other research programs at the state level and in foundation-funded research. We women led the way. We have a voice and we're out of estrogen, so listen up!

My work on the Scientific Peer Review Panel was challenging and exciting. First, it fed the science-hungry part of me that had not been so directly addressed since I left nursing. Second, reviewing proposals stretched me and taught me so many new things. My first time reviewing proposals was on the panel looking at molecular biology research. This was some heavy intellectual lifting! My main responsibility was to be able to read and understand the overall purpose and aim of the proposal and to comment on its relevance from my perspective as someone who had been through breast cancer and my knowledge of other survivors' experiences. All this reading and evaluating was going on in the isolation of my little screened porch in Chattanooga, Tennessee, where I sat surrounded by two Xerox boxes shipped to me by the DoD, containing over 50 proposals! I had another experienced consumer reviewer as my mentor, who calmed me down and helped me not to be overwhelmed by the sheer volume of the proposals. I also had access to the Executive Secretary of my review panel, who called periodically to be sure that I wasn't melting down. Elaine Hill had also served as a reviewer and offered me encouragement and practical tips on how to break down the review process.

I needed familiarity with all the proposals because I had an equal vote with the MD's and PhD's on my panel. I also had to write my own reviews on 17 of them, summarizing what each proposal was about, commenting on relevancy, raising any issues I wanted to, and making comments in other areas (if I had the knowledge or audacity to do so). Actually, several times my perspective as a breast cancer survivor has swayed the panel members' opinions. Of course, many times, they have also illuminated my understanding and influenced my final vote.

Reading through all the proposals was a great experience! I couldn't discuss any of the exciting ideas I was seeing in the proposals because they contained proprietary information. As I sat there, though, with my highlighter pen and a three-foot high stack of typed pages next to me, I was blown away to think that these fine minds were throwing their energies and expertise at breast cancer, to help people like me! Since I was working in the area of molecular biology, I had to adjust to and accept the fact that much of the basic science research would take a long time to get from the lab bench to the patient. Some of it was being conducted in yeast and fruit flies, for goodness sake, so vertebrates seemed a long way away in the distant future. But wasn't it wonderful that there was money to help understand breast cancer at its most basic foundations? There were so many interesting ideas and hypotheses. All of them had to be substantiated by existing scientific findings in order to be submitted for consideration. As I immersed myself in possibilities, I could only think about the quantum leaps that had been made in science and medicine because an observant scientist working on something over here just happened to notice something odd happening over there and thought, "Hmmmm... I wonder..." Voilá!! Penicillin, the double helix, smallpox vaccine, the recognition of AIDS, and on and on. I felt like I was being allowed to stand in a birthing room for breakthroughs.

After writing my reviews, I shipped the big boxes of hard copies back to Washington, DC and got ready to make my trip to sit on the review panel. I'll have to confess that the unreformed hippie part of me wondered how weird it was going to be to rub elbows with all this Army brass. Although we never ultimately followed through with this option, during the Viet Nam war, I'm the girl who once had immigration papers for Canada, when David and I had decided, "Hell, no! He won't go!" After we became Baha'is, we shifted our stance because Baha'is obey civil law. David was drafted, but served in a noncombatant role. We had endured his two years in the Army but I had retained my aversion to most things military.

I arrived at the DC suburb of Tyson's Corner, Virginia for

our review sessions and met scientists from every place imaginable, from the most famous research labs, people whose names had graced the pages of *Nature* and *Science*, not to mention prestigious medical journals on both sides of the Atlantic. I met oncologists and other clinicians who cared for patients daily and were also doing research. I met full-bird colonels and majors and captains in full uniform who were the warmest folks and the most passionate of all about breast cancer research and the work they were charged to be part of. In seconds, it was obvious that we were all definitely on the same team and these were hard-working, expert, sincerely motivated people. I was immediately drawn to Colonel Kenneth Bertram, who headed the program. His deep commitment to whatever made the best research possible, his respect and concern for breast cancer survivors, and his warm manner won me over quickly. I could easily relinquish my youthful "black or white" view of the Department of Defense.

Best of all, I met other breast cancer advocates who were on the front lines, just like me, who had their own stories and breast cancer work. There's no energy like the energy in a room full of breast cancer survivors. I made some good friends, friends I still have who know my heart and my life from a distance through email, until our paths cross again at some breast cancer conference. At the opening plenary session, one of my heroes, Fran Visco, spoke. She was the founder of the National Breast Cancer Coalition and is still intimately and crucially involved each year in securing Congressional funding for breast cancer research. Since the beginning of the program in 1992 through Fiscal Year 2005, $1.8 billion has been directed to breast cancer research.

There were 20 review panels going on simultaneously. Serving on my panel as a "virgin" was a little daunting at first, but as we all introduced ourselves and the scientists heard us briefly tell our stories as breast cancer survivors, I could feel the shift in the room.

I experienced respect and welcome. There seemed to be a softening and a falling away of any academic posturing. Our presence was a reminder of why these scientists worked so hard every day and a reminder that what they did as researchers really mattered.

One evening, three panels got together and went to a great Chinese restaurant. People whom I had thought would be dour, ivory tower scientists got up and told some of the worst jokes I've ever heard. We had a marvelous time.

The entire experience was one of the best of my life, and I was incredibly lucky to be able to repeat it. I was honored to participate on DoD panels over the next five years. I reviewed hundreds of proposals in the areas of cell biology, pathobiology, and molecular genetics, as well as "Innovator" proposals, clinical translation proposals, and those supporting Historically Black Colleges and Universities (HBCU's) to help them begin or strengthen their breast cancer research programs in partnership with established research facilities.

What about the girl with the hippie heart who had her doubts about consorting with the military? I'm now a convert. I can't imagine any government institution doing a better job of administering this program with more energy, integrity, efficiency, and passion than the U.S. Army. It was my privilege.

You are so weak. Give up to grace.
The ocean takes care of each wave
till it gets to shore.
You need more help than you know.
You're trying to live your life in open scaffolding.

- Rumi

Chapter 8

My work at Y-ME continued to be both gratifying and difficult. In 1999, I was approaching the five-year mark since my cancer
diagnosis. My breast reconstruction was complete. I was entering
my final year of taking Tamoxifen, the estrogen blocker prescribed
at that time to most postmenopausal women to help stave off recurrence. I was getting restless to move beyond breast cancer. In my
personal life, other than the daily reminder of the Tamoxifen tablet,
life was feeling more normal at last.

Working 40 hours a week in breast cancer focused me every day on my own health. I began to see a toll taken on my family, too. Hearing about women in crisis, even peripherally, kept
them stirred up and uncertain about my health. Steve's comment
about being forced to watch a car wreck over and over haunted
me. I was the one watching the car wrecks every day and I was
beginning to fray.

In the early autumn of 1999, I decided that it was time to
leave Y-ME. I talked with Elaine Hill about my decision. I felt sorry

to leave work that was meaningful every second of every day, but I was becoming convinced that the emotional expense was not good for me and therefore ultimately not good for Y-ME. As both my boss and my friend, she understood. I left Y-ME at the end of January 2000 and began my new job on February 1 in the Development Office of another non-profit, Family and Children's Services of Chattanooga (now Partnership for Families, Children and Adults).

In our own family, Hollin was in the full throes of adolescent rebellion. It was a very difficult time that would span several years. On the bright side, Steve's son Chris had moved back to Chattanooga and had become engaged to a wonderful woman. He was opening a new restaurant that would feature murder mysteries in a dinner theater format. Chris and Jennifer planned to marry in mid-June and open the restaurant several days after that. My relationship with Steve's daughter, Laura, had also become close and was a source of happiness and sustenance to me.

My own health was generally good, but in April, I noticed a sore place just to the left of my old mastectomy scar, directly over the breastbone. I felt unsettled by it and saw my surgeon, Laura Witherspoon. She did an ultrasound and saw nothing. Going back for follow-up in the early summer, I still complained of tenderness in that spot. She ordered blood work and a bone scan, which still showed nothing.

Summer brought the flurry of Chris's wedding and the whole family pitching in to help with the opening and staffing of Hampton's Vaudeville Café. That summer and into the fall, after work I went to the café to help as the dishwasher. Lifting racks of dishes and glasses out of the steaming dishwasher, I noticed that the sore place over my breastbone was larger and more painful, aggravated by exercise. In late summer, Dr. Witherspoon did a needle biopsy of the area, which came back negative.

By early October, I began to notice that the sore place even hurt when people hugged me. I called Dr. Witherspoon again. When we met, she suggested that we do an open biopsy to rule out anything serious, once and for all. She scheduled my procedure for late October, and I came through the minor surgery without a hitch. Post-op, Dr. Witherspoon reassured Steve that what she had excised looked like just fat and scar tissue. That was on a Friday.

Monday, Steve and I met at Rembrandt's Coffee House, one of our favorite places in Chattanooga's Bluff View Art District. We savored lunch and the gorgeous autumn weather, talking about possibilities for when we could retire. Steve dropped me off back at the agency, and I went to my office and checked my voicemail. I broke into a sweat as I heard Dr. Witherspoon's carefully measured words, asking me to call her. I did.

Voicemail

We sat and talked of our retirement,
    dreaming over after-lunch coffee
    in the gold of a fall afternoon,
    the little bandage from my biopsy still on my chest,
    but our hearts filled with reassurance that all was well.
When I returned to my office
    the carefully-modulated voice
    of my surgeon said to call her immediately,
and I knew that the house of my future
had been blasted to matchsticks.

Dr. Witherspoon's voice came on the line. "I'm so sorry, Debbi," she began, a catch in her own voice. "The pathology report just came back and it shows a 4 millimeter area of lobular breast cancer. Could you come to the office now so that we can talk over what's next?"

I felt numb. I was sleepwalking, disembodied. This couldn't be real. I called Steve and he began driving back toward my office. I went through the halls, and walked straight into my boss's office. "My cancer's back," I sobbed. Farrell Cooper had himself had cancer years before, and I couldn't have had a more understanding friend at that moment. He hugged me and said, "We'll do whatever you need us to do. Go find out what's next and just let me know."

Steve picked me up. Everything seemed sharp-edged and surreal. He kissed me hello and touched me often as we drove the ten minutes to Dr. Witherspoon's office. His jaw was set and I could see that he was struggling for control, too. When we arrived, the nurse quickly escorted us into the doctor's office. Dr. Witherspoon came in and hugged each of us. Laura Witherspoon was not only my surgeon, but had served on my Board of Directors at Y-ME. Steve and I had danced at her 40th birthday party. This was hard for all of us. Her own eyes filled with tears. "I am so sorry about this news. I had absolutely no reason to doubt that everything was normal in the tissue that I removed or I would not have offered you reassurance the other day." We knew that. It was just one of those things.

"So, what's next?" I asked.

Dr. Witherspoon smiled gently. "Now begins the unpleasant cascade of medical decisions and treatment. I've made an appointment with Frank Kimsey, the radiation oncologist, for tomorrow morning. I've also called your oncologist, Dr. Johnson, to let him know this news. We'll all confer. Radiation is definitely in the picture. Since this is a small area, Dr. Johnson may or may not feel that chemotherapy is indicated." She paused. "Surgically speaking, we'll need to take your implant out on the right. Radiation therapy will cause scarring and will compromise your reconstruction on that side."

I was stunned. I'd have to lose my new breast on the right? The force of my grief bulldozed me. "Could I have Dr. von Werssowetz involved in that process, in case there is a chance later to rebuild?" I asked through tears.

"Of course," she answered. "Do you want me to call him for you?"

"I don't mind calling him," I said. "I'll probably have questions for him anyway. I know that you'll need to talk with him for scheduling, though."

Dr. Witherspoon called Dr. Von and he agreed to be present for the surgery. It was scheduled for the next week. Steve and I left the office shattered and frightened.

At home, I tried to make sense out of the news. How could this have happened? I had been on Tamoxifen all that time. I had only been off it for a few months. I resented having cancer crowd my thoughts again. I didn't want it to run my life again! What had I done or not done that made the cancer come back? In a moment of superstition, I recalled that just weeks earlier, I had written an article about my breast cancer experience and for the first time had said, "I had breast cancer" rather than "I have breast cancer." Steve had even pointed this out to me jubilantly, as a sign of my being done with it.

Larceny

Like the sight of a doorknob turning
The stalker pursues me
     teasing
         waiting patiently.
I called him to me.
I used the past tense to refer to my cancer
and within weeks

was on the O.R. schedule for an open biopsy
that showed the invader back again,
with roots sunk down deep.

Cancer is a thief
robbing me of my fragile security
and sometimes stealing my self,
leaving me with a ransacked identity.

The possibility of spread to other organs loomed much larger, too. We met with Dr. Johnson, who had cared for me since I began working for Y-ME. He was inclined to suggest at least some chemotherapy. The next diagnostic steps included CT scans, MRI's, and a bone scan. The results of those tests could make the news even worse.

As I lay on different exam tables over the next several days with a variety of radioactive isotopes zinging through my veins, I was aware that my fate and future were being traced in images onto the faces of computer screens. All we could do was wait. In some ways, I felt an odd sense of relief, as though I had been waiting for years for the other shoe to drop. The worst that I had feared had finally happened. The anticipation of that was gone. Its absence, however, made room for the next level of fear to bubble up. What if the cancer had spread to other organs?

Finally, we sat in a room at Dr. Johnson's office, waiting to hear the results of all the tests. Steve nervously read an old *Time* magazine from back to front. I heard Dr. Johnson's steps in the hallway. I heard the swish of papers as he took my chart out of the file holder on the door. I held my breath. He opened the door. Before he even got across the threshold, he said, "All the scans were negative. There's no evidence of metastases in any organs anywhere."

With a strangled sob, Steve's face crumpled into tears. I felt my eyes fill and a weight lift off me. What a reprieve! Just a little chest wall recurrence! Good news! I laughed in relief and with an awareness of the crazy irony, the goofy logic of cancer. Where the news of a chest wall recurrence had brought us to our knees just a week before, now we were all giving each other high fives!

Dr. Johnson outlined the plan. Dr. Kimsey confirmed that my surgeons would need to go back in to remove the implant. While I was under anesthesia, Dr. Witherspoon would also insert a port-a-cath, a large permanent IV that is placed in the big subclavian vein just under the collarbone. For delivering the course of chemo-therapy that Dr. Johnson was proposing to give me, this would be the safest and most convenient route. Removing the breast implant was a simple procedure. The surgeons would open the area near my old scar, remove my implant, and take a larger tissue sample while they were there. That would be it and it wouldn't take long, not more than an hour.

Chapter 9

The day of the surgery arrived. Steve sat in the surgical waiting area. One hour stretched into two and then two into three and then three into four. The surgery was taking a long time because when the doctor removed the implant, a large area in the chest wall was now exposed and was riddled with cancer.

Dr. Witherspoon worked her way out concentrically and methodically, sending off tissue sample after tissue sample to try to get clean margins. At one point, apparently, the pathologist who had been examining the samples of my cancer sent to him from surgery suited up and came into the operating room to see what was going on.

In the recovery area, Dr. Witherspoon talked to both of us, saying that what we had thought was a 4-millimeter area turned out to be more like 4 by 6 centimeters and extended downward through the chest muscle sometimes as deeply as 3 centimeters, adhering to the breastbone. She said, "I was never able to get clean margins along the area I was excising. I marked the area with clips so that Dr. Kimsey will know where I was working when he does your radiation therapy planning. I did finally go out toward your armpit and took a sample and it was clean. The size of this mass changes the picture. I'm sure that Dr. Johnson will want to meet with you as soon as possible to revisit his plan for systemic chemotherapy." She was tender with us and concerned.

In the through-the-looking-glass world of cancer, good news and bad news are relative and fluid. We had been devastated about the 4-millimeter lesion. We had been elated by clean scans. Now we were facing a regional recurrence the size of a pork chop. Despite that awful news, we realized how fortunate we were that the open biopsy had hit this little tail of the larger tumor and that a good pathologist had found it, despite the fact that on gross examination, the tissue had appeared to be fat and scar tissue. My overriding feeling was just plain lucky.

Where there had evidently been some inter-specialty debate as to whether chemotherapy was really needed, there was no question now. The expanded plan that Dr. Johnson outlined for us was that after a course of Adriamycin and Cytoxan and then radiation therapy to the chest wall daily for five weeks, he would then come back around with Taxotere, another chemotherapy drug, completing my treatment around June.

In between appointments that filled the squares of my calendar, I tried to deal with this new reality that had been imposed on me. One thing I found was that I was more shaken by the loss of my reconstructed breast than I had ever been by my first two mastectomies. To me, this was a third mastectomy and the loss of a breast that I had chosen to have. I had lost a powerful symbol of my wellness. In addition to the grief I felt, I had to adjust to the way that I looked, with my loose skin, the pitiful little deflated pocket that had once contained the implant, and the bedraggled nipple tattoo. Where being a bilateral mastectomy had looked a little strange, I had not felt disfigured. The remnant of my reconstructed right breast looked bizarre, but there was nothing to be done for it. Until I completed radiation therapy sometime in the spring and healed from that, I couldn't shop for a breast prosthesis to even me up in how my clothing fit me.

Once again, I was getting an education about my reality. My physical body was being literally chipped away. I reminded myself that it was just a vessel, something to which my soul was lightly attached. I had to focus on what made me myself, what part I could nurture and try to develop. It was a double-edged process, allowing myself to grieve for what I had physically lost so that I could more cleanly and fully step towards my spirit. I realized that I couldn't do one without the other. If I blocked the sadness, it would build a wall that kept me from my true self.

I had a routine test to be sure that my heart could withstand Adriamycin, which occasionally can damage heart muscle. Dr. Johnson decided to use a portable infusion pump about the size of a small radio that I would wear so that he could give me the Adriamycin over three days. He was safeguarding my heart since while normal, test findings for how my heart was pumping were on the low side of normal.

I had my first treatment the day before Thanksgiving, four days after my surgery. We stocked up on Jell-O and yogurt, custard and crackers, Cokes and ginger ale, not knowing if I would be sick to the stomach from the chemotherapy. Steve and I spent Thanksgiving that year piled up together on our fold-out couch in front of the fireplace, watching football and eating soft, bland food, my infusion pump hanging from my waist and whirring like a little camera advancing film as it measured and pumped my medicine, minute by minute. I did pretty well, using the oral medication that Dr. Johnson had prescribed to prevent nausea to reinforce what the nurses had given me by IV. Because of the holiday weekend, a home health nurse came out the day after Thanksgiving and, donning full biohazard attire, removed my pump and disposed of the tubing and needle. I felt like a toxic waste dump. If this stuff had to be disposed of like this, what was it doing inside me? It was a graphic reminder that basically I was getting poison – proven, effective poison, but still poison.

I went from appointment to appointment and back and forth to work, juggling around the side effects of the chemo and the scheduling challenges imposed by treatment. Just under my skin, I was always aware that I was angry about this damned disease returning, despite all the aggressive and excessive treatment I had thrown at it the first time around. I was furious that this could have happened again and furious was where I stayed for several months.

Dance

This second time around
         is not so terror-filled.
I know this cancer-dance
and most of its steps.
The one that leads me
will dance me into the ground.
My days are marked by
         appointments
         tests
         treatments
         blood work,
My hours by medication,
Infusion pump readings.

I'll dance this dance
because I have no choice,
but I hate it,
and my anger burns
my footprints into the floor.

With this chemo regimen, for the first time I would lose all my hair. Anticipating that, I did several things: got my hair cut even shorter than I usually wore it, bought a wig, and had a family portrait taken before my hair fell out. The portrait was taken in the gardens at the Chattanooga Choo Choo, the evening before hair began falling out by the handful, into my face and my food with every turn of my head, right on schedule on day 13 after my first treatment with Adriamycin.

Until it happened to me, I had believed that you could soften the shock of losing all your hair. Yes, cutting your hair shorter means that you only have inch-long wads of it coming out in your hands when you shampoo, instead of foot-long strands. The end result still buckled my knees the first time I saw myself in the mirror.

My family was a huge help in meeting this head-on with me, trying to normalize the situation as much as possible. It didn't take long for me to decide that I just wanted my head shaved rather than to go through several days of picking hair out of my eyes and mouth and watching clumps of it fall on my pillow, in the shower, and onto my clothes. The evening we finally decided to completely shave my head, the family was there, including Laura and my oldest grandchildren, Jesseca and Colby.

Steve had said he would shave me. Hollin, who had been very avoidant of everything to do with this recurrence, surprised me by asking to cut my hair super short before Steve applied the razor to me. It was an intimate act on her part and I felt that to get in as close as she had to signaled some acceptance of our new circumstances.

I sat in our kitchen, perched on a chair, with a sheet on the floor under me. Laura got me a stuffed animal to hold and gave me loving encouragement. Jesse and Colby were in and out of the kitchen, curious but not anxious.

After both Hollin and Steve had finished, Hollin said, "Mom! You look just like Granddad Lang!" I went into the bathroom to look in the mirror for the first time.

Stripped

Bald before the mirror, I look frailer without hair.
I see my father
> *and all the Langs before me*
> *gazing back at me.*
I'm stunned.
I thought I resembled my mother
> *but stripped to my cranium,*
> *pale and sick from chemo,*
I could pass for my eighty-six-year-old father's sister –
Not his late-in-life daughter.

I looked so much sicker suddenly. Was it only a little over two months before that I had felt comfortable in my own skin? This person in the mirror looked like a stranger to me.

Steve took a series of portraits of me during that time that now, years later, seem to have a stark, defiant beauty. One time he said to me that I looked "like an extraterrestrial princess." Some friends around the country who had heard that I was in treatment again and who had been through this themselves sent their own bald pictures. It really helped as I adjusted to being bald.

I did wear my wig. I didn't always want to have to explain my looks. Each morning it was enough of an effort to piece myself together with wig, fiberfill in my empty bra cup, and make-up to rosy up my anemic cheeks and lips. Some days it felt like Halloween. Most days, it was just the new "normal." Pulling on a wig and not having to fix my hair meant an extra half hour of sleep in the morning. There were some payoffs.

I tried to keep as normal a schedule as possible. Each round of chemo produced slightly more severe side effects, from dropping blood counts to nausea that was about the grade of morning sickness. I worked through most of this time, which was essential for my mental health.

Steve and I also had a regular paying job as musicians on Saturday evenings at a large Mexican restaurant in Dalton, Georgia. Playing out was great for my head and my heart. The only concession I made was that on the day after my chemo, I ordered a simple plate of refried beans instead of my usual chicken enchilada with tomatillo salsa and a side of guacamole.

Despite going through all the motions of maintaining a normal life, I felt so stuck in my anger. It was freeing to give up trying to be the poster child for survivorship, but I didn't want to have to fuel that decision with anger. I felt so betrayed by my body. I had prayed. I had railed at Fate. I had whined. Still the anger simmered in me. When I really didn't know what else to do and felt helpless to move past being so angry, a friend gave me a copy of *My Grandfather's Blessings*, a book by Rachel Naomi Remen. It changed my life. The book combines stories and lessons learned early in her life from her grandfather, who was a rabbi, with stories of her work with people facing life-threatening disease (mostly cancer). For me, in addition to her views on how each of us can become a blessing, the core of the book seemed to speak to me about finding meaning in suffering.

The words of Remen's book and the stories of others who had struggled with difficulties drove me back to the roots and writings of my own faith. If I truly believed that my reality was spiritual and that tests and suffering could strengthen and open me more fully to life and loving, then I had to trust this process. There is a phrase in one of the Baha'i prayers, talking about how challenges can be the fodder for drawing closer to God and to one's own spiritual reality. It says, "…the food of them that haste to meet Thee is the fragments of their broken hearts."

I'm convinced that I needed, what we call in the South, a "big whup upside the head" to get my attention. My personal trials and the ongoing challenges of breast cancer were my call to action, and I'm very grateful. If this was what my life was going to be, I had to have faith that my job was to lean into the gale-force winds of it all and know that they would take me where I was supposed to go.

As I approached the last of my four rounds of Adriamycin and Cytoxan, I found myself with a growing aversion to my doctor's office and to submitting to chemo. Always tough in the past and able to set my jaw and get through it, now I winced even at simple finger-sticks for the weekly blood work. I stuck my finger out for the technician, but turned my head to hide the tears that stood in my eyes. I got my chemotherapy but I dreaded the purple fog of drugs and intrusive nausea that would persist for about two weeks out of the three. Then, when I'd finally be feeling physically better the last week before the next treatment, my blood counts would bottom out. I'd be pooped from anemia and forbidden to do anything fun or social outside of home for fear of infection. I just finally had to give myself over to the fact that I had no choice in this matter.

Breast cancer was relentlessly and sometimes ruthlessly teaching me that there was only one thing in my life that I could have choice over, that I could control: how I respond to this disease. To get internal healing, I had to believe that I would be given the capacity to transcend my physical circumstances. Once I had that knowledge deep inside me, my anger evaporated and a peace came over me.

An interesting by-product of this shift was that I became less and less self-conscious about my baldness, and even occasionally whipped off the wig if I had a particularly strong hot flash. As we moved through winter and I adjusted to the temperature changes that go with no hair, I began to wear my wig less often at home.

During this time, friends drowned us in their love. A girlfriend coordinated everyone's cooking and other help, to ensure that we had a steady inflow of home-cooked meals and not periods when there was either nothing to fall back on or too much food hanging over the shelves of the fridge and freezer. Friends whose names I'll never know chipped in and paid for a housekeeper to come twice a month to rescue me from total slovenliness and restore order to my home. Everyone's kindness was overwhelming. I was beginning to learn to accept and to allow people to serve and help in these ways.

I also had at least one friend with me for every chemo treatment, as well as Steve for at least part of each treatment. This was no small sacrifice for friends to arrange; it took several hours for me to get the drugs. On the last treatment, I had only Steve with me and tired as I was by then, it was wonderful to be able just to lean back and close my eyes when I needed to. We also played cribbage through most of the last treatment, to pass the time. Before we went for my treatment, I called him to task. When I reminded him to bring the cribbage board, I also cautioned my sometimes-salty husband that we'd be among other patients in this Catholic hospital. I said, "Steve, you know that if you get a bad cribbage hand, you can't be swearing about it!"

He looked at me with a twinkle in his eye and said, "Oh! I understand! Does that also mean that in that room full of people taking chemotherapy that if you get a good hand, I can't call you a lucky shit?"

I felt blessed once again with the keen awareness of the sweetness of life and the simple things around me, and this time that awareness stuck. I moved toward my radiation therapy tired but calm, grateful to be a third of the way through my treatments.

Last year, I gazed at the fire.
This year I'm burnt kabob.

- Rumi

Chapter 10

Mid-February of 2001, it was time to start my radiation therapy. Simple-minded me, I was glad to get on with this part of my treatment. I thought I understood (and believed) how it worked: there was still cancer in my chest, the doctor would aim radiation directly at the cancer, and radiation kills cancer. I had lots of faith in that. Dr. Kimsey planned to irradiate not only the center of my chest where the cancer still was, but also several inches to the left of the midline, down to the bottom of the ribs, over to under my right arm, and up toward my jaw line on the right. This was to include any region where cancer cells might be setting up housekeeping. He promised me what he euphemistically called "a brisk skin reaction." I later found out just what that meant.

The day we did my radiation planning, I was lying on the table and the doctor was working on me, surveying my chest after looking at the CT scans. Radiation therapy is very precise, and this planning session would set everything up for the next six weeks. Dr. Kimsey was wielding a great, broad-nibbed, orange permanent marker. With one eye, I was watching him as he boldly marked off my chest with certitude and even gusto. With the other eye, I was watching the clock, making sure that I'd have time to make it to a noon commitment for work to help promote a big fund-raising event. As he looped the marker across my neck, up under my right ear and back down in a nice parabola of bright orange, I started giggling. He grinned and asked, "Am I tickling you?"

"No," I answered. "I've just got to go on Channel 9 at noon today to promote our big auction!"

Special lead blocks were custom made to target the radiation beams to the areas we needed to go after and to protect the tissue we didn't want to damage. After the planning, I went through a simulation of the treatment, to be sure that all the blocks and settings were just right. I would soon be ready to start my treatments.

One of the hardest aspects of this round of chemotherapy was the bone-crushing fatigue. I'm normally an energetic person, but I found myself at the end of the workday literally shedding clothes as I arrived home so that I could fall in bed for a few hours to recover enough energy to enjoy my family in the evening and to do the things I needed to do outside of work. Cancer fatigue is in a category all by itself. I found it to be unremitting and unrelieved, even by sleep. The patient literature about radiation therapy promised "progressive and cumulative fatigue." If I was starting radiation already so tired, I tried to imagine how I would be at the end of radiation! Then I still had a couple more months of chemo to go. I reminded myself for the hundred thousandth time, "One day at a time."

On my first day of radiation treatment, I arrived and got into my hospital gown. The technician led me into the treatment room where she had me lie down on a narrow metal platform that must have been precooled to about 36 degrees. She opened my gown to expose three-quarters of my chest and then asked me to relax and not move. I needed to lie there like a sack of flour and let her position my body to line me up with the laser crosshairs projected across my chest. My head was stabilized in a little, hard, uncomfortable headrest. I thought of scenes from *Shogun*, with the hardy Japanese lying on mats on the floor with a block for a pillow. Maybe Samurai warrior imagery was a good thing to hang onto.

As the tech left the room, she said, "We're taking an X-ray first. A light on the wall will go on. Lie still. After the X-ray, you'll see the light go on again for your treatment. I'll come back in and we'll change positions to get the next area treated, too."

She left the room and I heard the big lead door shut. I really had no idea what to expect. I knew that everything was carefully programmed into a computer, but this was an exercise in trust, for sure. I saw the little light saying "Beam is On" blink for a fraction of a second as my chest X-ray was taken. Then about a minute later, the light went back on, and stayed on. There was no feeling and not much sound, except the hum of the machine and the lighted sign on the wall. I counted to 45. Finally, it went off.

Radiation Therapy

I am carefully wedged into position
on the gantry
Paperweighted down by lead blocks
that define the bad and protect the good,
Creating a bordered target for the rays of radiation
shielding the essentials, like my heart,
From cosmic sizzle.
Positioned carefully
by degrees and millimeters,
I am locked in place.

The techs scurry for safety
and slam the ponderous door.
I am sealed in, secure as a bank vault,
My only companion
The eerie hum of the linear accelerator
and the light saying
Radiation on

on

on.

I count the seconds
and hope they got it right.

From the time that I stepped into the room, the whole treatment took about 10 minutes, about eight of which were spent positioning the platform and me. Going every weekday became a routine. Skin care was a priority. I was not to use regular soaps or deodorant on the treatment side. As the weeks progressed, my skin got pinker and pinker. There was a nice little tint of rose that fell precisely within the marked area of my treatment field. Then, toward the end of the fifth treatment week, I awoke one morning with some pain and the skin looking like a mega-sun-burn. It was unpleasant, but bearable. The techs and nurses did not seem surprised.

Over the weekend, however, I developed tenderness across my chest and under my arm that was severe enough that I could not comfortably put my right arm down against my side. It felt like a big abscess. The skin looked really damaged, swollen and ruby red. I was in knee-walking pain but thought, I'm just being a big baby. Maybe it's just because I'm sick of all of this.

I went for my regular appointment on Monday with Dr.

Kimsey. He took one look at my chest and pulled out a prescription pad. "Have you been taking anything for pain?"

"Tylenol," I answered, "but it's not doing much."

He wrote me a prescription for Oxycontin and another one for Percodan. "Take the Oxycontin regularly," he told me. "Don't just stop taking it abruptly once you've started, either. We'll need to taper you off it in a few weeks. You have a radiation burn and cellulitis. I know it really hurts, but we'll get you healed up. I'm also prescribing Silvadene cream for the burn. We're still going to do the booster treatments at a higher dose of radiation next week. We'll keep a close eye on your skin. This is going to get worse for a few weeks before it gets better. Preventing infection is going to be the most important, so I'm also putting you on an antibiotic. Take the Oxycontin as I'm prescribing it, and use the Percodan for any breakthrough pain."

I wasn't just being a baby! This was serious pain. I wondered to myself why it was that, at nearly 50 years old, I still needed someone else to validate what my own senses were telling me. I needed permission from someone outside of myself to hurt or feel bad. Tears filled my eyes as I walked down the hall to see my oncologist for my regular appointment with him.

When Dr. Johnson saw my chest, he drew his breath in sharply, took out his prescription pad, and began writing "Oxycon..."

"Dr. Kimsey just saw me," I interrupted him. "I've got a prescription for Oxycontin and Percodan from him."

"Well, don't hesitate to take it," he said. "We'll keep a close eye on your blood counts, too, to be sure you don't get an infection. If you run a fever, we'll admit you to the hospital. It may take a good month to get you completely healed up. If we need to delay your chemo with Taxotere, don't worry. We'll just wait until you are completely healed."

I spent the next three weeks wearing drawstring pants and

oversized tee shirts that I changed three times a day, each time Steve applied the Silvadene cream. He was a great nurse, faithfully taking care of the burn. I showered each time before the next slathering with Silvadene, the water washing the debris away.

I worked at my job about six hours a day most of this time. I was up against a deadline for core funding for our agency of about $3,000,000 over the next three years, so I needed to work. The only thing that enabled me to function was the Oxycontin. Because it is a time-released narcotic, I got good pain relief and wasn't gorked out by it. I hid out in my office most of this time in my lovely tee shirt ensembles, but I got the work done.

Radiation Burn

After five weeks of radiation therapy
that imparted the pink blush of a sunburn
I awake to purple pain
and a burgundy chest
that, overnight, looks like I was caught in a house-fire.
Radiation burn.
The days become centered around soothing Silvadene cream
and staying ahead of the pain,
a constant deep throb over three square feet of my skin,
which hangs in strips where burn blisters have burst.
I spend three weeks in tee shirts,
blessing my husband for his courageous, constant care
to this tissue-strewn disaster area.
I am thankful for the Oxycontin that delivers me
sustains me

enables me to function
And I curse the short-sighted, ill-informed feds
who would take this narcotic miracle off the market
because last year 100 addicts — who could choose life —
o.d.'ed on it
instead of some other drug of choice.

Dr. Kimsey warned me that the burn would continue to worsen after the radiation treatments were over, peaking about two weeks afterwards. He was right. Gradually, the swelling began to go down, and new pink healthy skin appeared. The pain diminished and finally, Dr. Kimsey began weaning me off the Oxycontin. By the third week in April, about two weeks ahead of schedule (thanks to Steve's great nursing care), I was healed enough to begin the next course of chemo. This was the home stretch.

Taxotere was not as challenging an experience for me as Adriamycin and Cytoxan had been. I had some flu-like symptoms, some numbness and tingling in my feet and pain in my toes, and some nail changes, but I had no nausea. I also had an odd but not uncommon phenomenon called "radiation recall." One morning several weeks into taking the Taxotere, I awoke with the same pain and feeling of heat that had characterized my radiation burn. I cautiously looked down at my chest, expecting to find it blistered again. The new pink skin was there, smooth and without blisters, but it was swollen and looked lightly sunburned. I hurt all the way down into my muscles, just like at the height of my radiation burn.

I called Dr. Kimsey and he explained that this effect occasionally happens when certain chemotherapy drugs are given after radiation treatment. What an odd effect! I thought. How could my own cells remember? It seemed like some strange post-hypnotic suggestion, activated within some primitive consciousness in the cell. I remembered how the physiologic as well as the psychological side of post traumatic stress disorder can be triggered by a sensory moment or memory, or even by an anniversary date of an event on the calendar. How little we truly understand of the complex relationships within us, messages conveyed by our souls and psyches and whispered cell to cell. Dr. Kimsey put me back on the Oxycontin for several more weeks. The swelling and pain in the area gradually resolved and I never experienced this again.

One aspect of taking Taxotere that was bothersome was taking Decadron, a powerful steroid, around the time of treatment to lessen the chance of an allergic reaction. The steroids made me very edgy emotionally, snappish and irritable. Steve and Hollin took this gripiness with humor, commenting to each other, "Mom's coming off the Decadron. Head for the hills!" as they anticipated my grumpy days.

In May, the local Y-ME chapter began offering a resource for women with advanced or recurrent breast cancer that has been a vital source of support for me ever since. Two licensed clinical social workers agreed to co-facilitate a therapy group for those of us coping with metastatic disease. I remember the first meeting, when six of us gathered on a balmy day, warm enough to wear sandals. Every single one of us had our big toes bandaged, to hide the unsightly nail changes from chemo. We all pointed at each other's feet, laughed and asked, almost in unison, "Taxotere or Taxol?" Already our common experience was apparent.

This community of women, who agreed to be there for one another for the long haul, has provided a unique and irreplaceable haven for me. I feel totally safe in that group, able to talk about absolutely everything without feeling guarded or as though I need to protect anyone from hard truths. It's not all grim, by any means. We really do laugh a lot. We engage in some of the most outrageous gallows humor, joking about things that we probably wouldn't dare to speak aloud anywhere else. Over the years, we've had members die. That hasn't been easy, but the sisterhood in that room and the depth and realness of the relationships forged there are among the richest in my whole life. Group members provide a level of trust and commitment that has eased what, for me, has been a hard and sometimes lonely journey. We've had members from 29 years old to nearly 70. I am awed and inspired by each one every time I'm with them. I've learned so much about living from these women.

June 14, 2001 was my last treatment with Taxotere. I had been fortunate to come through all of my chemo and radiation and low blood counts without as much as a cold. When the oncology nurse "unplugged" me from the last IV of chemo, I thought Yeeaaa! I'm home free! Of course, I wasn't thinking about the next three weeks of the effects of chemo... I had low blood counts the second week and began running fever. The doctor put me on oral antibiotics, but the fever persisted, and I developed a cough. I called the nurse in his office when I was returning for blood work the following week, and she said for me to come back to the treatment room once I had my blood count results. The white counts had dropped even more, edging toward 1000 (normal counts are 4,000 – 11,000). She listened to my chest and said that I had diminished breath sounds. When she put me in an exam room for the doctor to see me, she patted me and said, "I can just about guarantee you that Dr. Johnson will admit you to the hospital. Do you want me to call your husband?"

I was still dubious, but when the doctor examined me, he said, "You've got pneumonia and you're not leaving here. Let me call admitting and you can hand-carry my orders to the oncology floor. "

I guess I had taken all of this pretty much in stride until I got to my room, then the serious activity began. This really was treated as a medical emergency. I was hustled into the bed. Nurses scrubbed up with Betadine before touching me, hooked me up to IV's quickly, and drew blood and blood cultures again and again. The nurses posted signs saying "neutropenia precautions." Everyone had to take extra care to protect me from any infectious threat because of my low blood counts. All food had to be cooked – no fruit, no raw veggies. Anyone visiting had to wash up with Betadine before coming near me. My grandchildren couldn't come in the room because the rule against children under 12 visiting was being strictly enforced. When I went down for my chest x-ray, I had to wear a facemask. While it was to protect me, I saw visitors back away from me as I zipped through the halls in my wheelchair. I felt like Typhoid Mary.

Steve brought me beautiful, orangey-red roses in full, extravagant bloom when he came the day I was admitted, but I couldn't even have those because of the infection precautions. I had him stand in the doorway and let me "oooh" and "aahhhh" over them before he took them to the nurses' station, where he asked the nurses to give them to someone who didn't have any flowers and just to tell them they had a secret admirer!

For a little while as I lay there on the oncology floor, I felt scared and wondered, Is this the beginning of how it's going to be? Is this the beginning of the end? I looked out the window and wondered, Will this be my last view of the world? Once I settled into the fear and cried, I could let it go and focus on the fact that this was just pneumonia, not end-stage cancer.

Aside from the fact that this was a serious thing and I had alarmed my family quite a bit, the up-side of being in the hospital was that I slept and slept and slept – about 10 hours each night - and napped during the day. No one made any requests or demands of me for four days. Finally, on the fourth day, my fever stayed down and my blood counts were back over 2000, my chest was clear (although the cough persisted), and I could go home.

Chemotherapy and radiation are the best treatments we have to kill cancer, but they fundamentally and systematically undermine your health. Several months before, Steve had carefully counted out three weeks from my last treatment on the calendar, drawing a big, blue box around July 5, saying from that point forward, my body would be on the upswing, from my blood counts to all of my body systems, beginning to rebuild my health.

Steve's hope for my returning health presumed that everything was fine after all this treatment. The next step was the scans. Dr. Johnson ordered CT scans of the chest, abdomen and pelvis, bone scans, and blood work. Steve and I waited anxiously for the results and for our meeting with him. As Dr. Johnson went through each report, page by page, he read the conclusions, saying those sweet words, "negative" and "no evidence of..." I was in full remission!

We realized that we had really been holding our breaths for a year and a half, since I first felt that sore place over my breastbone. What a relief to breathe again.

The light changes.
I need more grace
than I thought.

- Rumi

Chapter 11

While the weight of active breast cancer had been lifted from me with the completion of my treatments and the good test results, it seemed that the fallout of breast cancer continued to rain down. This was a time of emotional tests. My relationship with Hollin was at its ebb. She was so angry with me, for everything, and it leaked out everywhere. She had opted for every kind of acting out that an adolescent could do. I felt helpless in the face of her scorn. We had a knockdown, drag-out argument at the end of May that ultimately led to our beginning counseling together, where we worked for over five months to rebuild. It was very hard work. I had entered counseling with her, steeled for her to use it to slam me over the head with her anger and resentment. Instead, I was amazed and awed by her courage, honesty, and willingness to face hard things together. I was so proud of her. We did some hard work together, both reaching deep inside to make changes. I had to let go of her, and that was very hard since she was just 17 and had not had a good track record of judgment or responsibility. I learned, however, that if I continued to hold on as tightly as my fear inclined me to do, I was going to lose her, and we were going down together.

Steve and I had many adjustments, too. After nearly a year of having structured our lives around my illness and cancer treatment, we had to realign ourselves, our time, and our expectations to a different calibration. I felt that I had let him down, getting sick again. So much had changed since we first were married. He had to live with the uncertainty that I faced. Together, we had to adjust to the physical changes in me, too.

One area that most doctors do not talk about with cancer patients is sexuality. I suppose that many are uncomfortable with the subject or don't feel that they have adequate expertise to advise their patients. Maybe they think, Well, at least you're alive, aren't you? For us, this was an area of huge adjustment.

Taking estrogen blockers, going through the rigors of chemo, losing my implant and feeling less confident about my looks, weight gain associated with the treatment -- all of these things affected my confidence. Physiologically, with no estrogen and even the little I could have been making in my adrenal glands blocked by drugs, it was as though my aging had occurred at an accelerated rate. Although I wasn't yet 50, my anatomy was like an old woman's. Having had a total hysterectomy and ovaries removed at age 39 and now taking the estrogen blockers, I realized that I was basically surgically and chemically castrated. I was like a car with the basic equipment for the ride still intact, but little or no fuel to turn the engine over.

The stresses and uncertainties of the cancer having returned compounded the problem. Our intimate life had always been a source of joy, freedom, and deep trust, reinforcing our connection to one another. Now, the mechanics were definitely affected and the elements of my desire were also compromised. We had to do a lot of frank talking and reassuring one another, checking out what we thought might be true and not just making assumptions. We each had to adjust our expectations. The changes I experienced were frustrating to me. I missed my old self. I have grieved this loss and it continues to be a source of sadness for me from time to time. Steve was patient but I know that the changes took a toll on him, too.

Quicksilver

Our passion for each other
        was always liquid
Quicksilver
        silk and ocean.
Our physical intimacy
        was a gift
        the distilled expression of our love
        essential
        elemental
        free.
My aging has been compressed into two months.
Sere and arid from chemotherapy
        and the abolition of the last small sources
            of estrogen,
I search my body for the traces of desire.
I am dry and dead.
Where once I was banked coals
        and you were tinder and pure oxygen,
I am now scattered ashes.
You patiently build a fire in the rain,
        tending me
With your hands, your mouth,
        your eyes, your words.

Through my primary care physician, I was referred to a local female gynecologist who was also an endocrinologist. She took time with me and referred me to a local female psychiatrist who specialized in menopausal issues and sexuality. These two wonderful physicians, who often collaborated, helped me tease out what factors were directly related to treatment, what were a result of depression, and what hormonal issues were at play. They helped me to fine-tune what we could. Steve and I slowly created a different kind of married life than we had before. It has required of us an increased level of trust. I experience a different kind of tenderness from him and towards him and an emotional intimacy of a deeper level than I thought possible. This area of our marriage requires frequent communication and reassurance. Patience and humor also help. I still miss me and probably always will.

In the fall of the year, everyone's lives changed with September 11 in New York City and Washington, DC. The magnitude of the acts of terrorism, the waste and destruction of innocent lives was impossible to take in fully. I returned over and over in my own memory to the Cuban missile crisis. The fear seemed familiar and yet different.

October, After 9/11

Crosshatch of contrail
Chevrons the autumn sky
The geese in October flight dark V's against the cloud-white slashes.
  This vapor shorthand verifies our heightened vigilance.
  Fighter jets streak above us,
  leaving their autographs in the morning air
  And we here on the ground get a prickle up our backs,
    sometimes looking over our shoulders

or sitting bolt upright in the night when sirens wail
where just last month
we might have turned softly in sleep
and drifted back to safety, warmth.
The sky's manuscript writes memories across my forehead.
I am transported back to the sounds
and smells of my childhood,
the feelings of being a schoolchild during the Bay of Pigs and
the Cuban Missile Crisis
thirty-nine years ago to the day
living in DC
knowing how few miles our home would be
from ground zero.
I smell the fall coats in the coat rack at school,
the fresh shellac on the wood,
the playground dust and chalky smell of the floor
as we huddled there – nose to the tile -
behind the inadequate shield of plywood and corkboard,
practicing for the Russians to bury us, indeed.
The air raid siren's mournful unrelenting song on Mondays at noon
My ten-year-old mind plotting how
I would run the mile home from school
through the familiar woods and across the creek
to mama
to mama
to mama.
My self-appointed detail at home was to check
the Clorox bottles full of drinking water in our basement
the cans of soup and the worn flannel blankets and pillows
the flashlights and batteries in our makeshift bomb shelter;
But even I knew at ten years old that ten miles away
from the fury of a nuclear bomb

was certain death
and probable incineration.
I had gazed in horror and fascination
at the ghostly perfect images of people
vaporized against the Hiroshima city walls
as I paged through Life *magazine's*
oversized book of photographs
of the Second World War.
We made air raid drills part of the typical school day
and tried to go on normally, with fear just under
our still summer-tanned skin.
Fear was a by-product of the weapons' threat
in those Cold War, H-bomb days.
Today, terror has tried to make its nest here as the primary weapon.
The threat of nuclear bombs, chemicals, or biological agents
stands in line behind
the potent artillery of undiluted fear.
We fight this schoolyard bully of an enemy
facing up to him
calling him what he is
yet sometimes changing our route home.

Steve and I had some important decisions to make about a trip out of the country that we had planned for December. The Baha'i World Center in Haifa, Israel had invited us for a nine-day pilgrimage. This is a very special and important time for members of my faith to pray in the holy places and to visit historic sites associated with our religion. We had looked forward eagerly to this time, but watched the political situation in the Middle East warily. In Israel itself, violence had increased during the autumn months, even in Haifa, which had an enviable reputation for its religiously diverse population living peacefully.

Back in May, when we had confirmed our intention to travel to Haifa, I had made a promise to myself. I had vowed that if I came through my treatment and was well enough to make my pilgrimage, I would walk from the foot of Mount Carmel, at the harbor in Haifa, up the terraced gardens of the Baha'i properties, that rise nearly a kilometer up the slopes of Mount Carmel. I would walk those steps to the golden-domed shrine that held the burial place of one of the prophet-founders of my faith and give thanks for the opportunity and health that brought me there.

As November turned to December, Steve and I had to decide whether to postpone our trip or go as planned. My closest friend at work, Helen (also a breast cancer survivor), helped me think it through. It finally came down to one bald question: was I more likely to die of metastatic breast cancer or in a bus bombing in Israel? We decided to go.

The time in Israel was so wonderful. On the last Friday in December, I sat at breakfast with an Iranian Baha'i woman from England. She asked what we were going to do the next day, when we had unstructured time from the busy pilgrimage schedule. I told her that I had recently been through treatment for a recurrence of breast cancer and that I had made a promise that if I were able to make my pilgrimage, I would walk up the terraces to the shrine. She grabbed my hands in hers. "I had breast cancer, too – last year! May I go with you?" She had not talked to another person who had been through breast cancer, and we shared so much with each other.

The next day, we met at the foot of Mount Carmel. Her two sons were with her, and Steve was with me. We set off together and slowly but steadily climbed the hundreds of steps up the steep slope, pausing to rest and enjoy the view of Haifa Bay and the pristine formal gardens. Side by side in the shrine, we offered our prayers of thanks and hope. It is one of the most treasured memories of my life.

The trip was incredible for Steve and me. There is no better way to increase closeness in a relationship than to "spiritualize" it. This time of pilgrimage, while very individual, was also a matrix for renewing our connection and solidifying the foundations of our marriage and love for one another. We finished the trip with five days in Greece, a leg of the trip that was a link for Steve with his heritage.

The next year, 2002, was full of blessedly normal life events and regular life concerns. Hollin continued to struggle with adolescent issues, but completed a GED course through her school system, which allowed her to walk across the graduation stage in cap and gown with her class, on time. It was a glorious day.

I turned 50 in 2002. Cancer had transformed my view of aging and birthdays. Where this milestone was difficult for many of my friends, I embraced it with gratitude. Birthdays? Bring 'em on! I want every single one of them that I can get.

In the summer of 2002, Steve's son Chris and his wife Jen had their first child, a son named Kistler. I loved and relished my older grandchildren thoroughly. I also had the added spiritual intimacy of being Jesseca and Colby's Sunday School teacher, watching their incredible minds and spirits bloom. But Kistler was the first grandchild that I got to know from the day that he was born. Having a brand new baby in the family was delicious!

I was fully savoring the wonderful family that life and circumstance had brought together. The chaos of my own family when I was growing up left me longing for a close family. I had always wanted three children. Fertility problems had made pregnancy difficult for me to achieve and sustain. I had miscarried one child before Hollin and lost another through an ectopic pregnancy after her. I took some comfort in the thought of those two little souls as my other two children, but still wished that Hollin had siblings. Then, I had the grace and gift of Steve's children, Chris and Laura, come into my life.

Given all the trials around Steve's and my relationship, a civil relationship with them would have been generous enough on their parts. But they are extraordinary people, committed to unity and willing to reach out and build relationships. From the beginning of our marriage, they embraced Hollin as their sister, a connection she needed so much and that comforted me. With honesty and commitment, over time they built their relationship with me. Their own mother and father raised them wonderfully, to be open-hearted, loving, fine people. They have kindly and sincerely made room for me in their lives. I regard them as family and am grateful that although I would never presume to edge into their mother's place or role with them in any way, God has blessed me with two other children in a unique relationship. Perhaps because our extended family members have worked hard at being a unified, functioning, loving blended family, we are able to accept each person's unique place without evident resentment or competition. We truly function on the belief that there is more than enough love to go around. The healing that goes with that has been a balm to me every single day. I'm grateful to have my long-held wish for an extended family that enjoys each other fulfilled so completely.

As I came out of a year of treatment, I was learning to put my breast cancer on the back burner between appointments, for the most part. Work, family, my marriage, and my other interests were finally able once again to take up a more appropriate and normal amount of space and energy in my life. There was still the challenge of checking in with the doctor every three months, waiting for an outside indicator of my health.

The medical appointments and scans every several months would preoccupy me with anxiety about what was happening below the surface of my life on a cellular level. I figured that since I was checked four times that year and I was concerned and hyper-aware of my breast cancer the week of the tests and then the week of my appointment with the doctor to find out the results of the tests, that was about 8 weeks out of the year. Still, it wasn't the constant low-level stress that was present during active treatment. It was like renewing a visa every three months. I'd go to the border, cross over into the land of uncertainty and then, if all was well, get my visa stamped and return to the land of the living for another three months.

Upon turning 18, Hollin had moved in with her longtime boyfriend. In the autumn of 2002, she became pregnant. Her relationship with her boyfriend began to deteriorate, and we weren't sure what she would do. At the time, it felt like I had to let go of the last threads of the dreams and hopes that I had for the life I had envisioned for her. I was grateful that she and I had spent the previous year restoring and rebuilding our relationship. We were able to enter this time with balance and respect in our dealings with each other. I was deeply concerned for her, especially for her finances and lack of readiness for more than a minimum wage job. I felt, however, that she could rise to the needs of a baby.

Early in 2003, I began experiencing a racing pulse, shortness of breath on exertion, and some episodes of profuse sweating. I was so fatigued, hardly able to climb the stairs at work. I saw my internist and we soon discovered that I had damage to my heart muscle, almost certainly from the Adriamycin I had taken in 2000-2001. I was also experiencing some problems with my heart rhythm and an average pulse of about 110. No wonder I was feeling weak and tired!

As we worked with a cardiologist to tackle the weakened heart muscle and the rhythm problems, it seemed odd to me to think that while I had been fairly certain that breast cancer would be the cause of my death, maybe my heart (or even some other thing) could do it.

Prom

Breast cancer has been my steady date
    In this school of hard lessons.
Recurrence has brought me to the prom
    the Big Dance,
        and I've been certain that cancer would take me home.
Held by him in close embrace on this dance floor,
    someone else cuts in.
My eager new partner
    leads me double-time around the floor
    until I am panting, pulse pounding.
He is my damaged heart,
    an unexpected suitor
    who vies for my attention
    and shows off his serious muscles.
His car is running in the parking lot
    and I don't know who is rushing me
    through the gym doors
    toward the darkness.

Sometimes, I felt so discouraged, when I felt like breast cancer was still running my life. There were periods when I felt that I was fighting for every day. I would get up each morning, and wash my scarred body, feeling the woody hardness of my chest where cancer, radiation, and multiple surgeries had left me bound down and misshapen. I'd pull on my bra and straighten my prosthesis. I'd choose clothing that would hide the protrusion of my port-a-cath, left in place "just in case." I'd gulp down my Arimidex to block any traces of estrogen and take the Wellbutrin to blunt the edge of depression that still seemed to sit on my shoulder. It was hard to get away from constant reminders. Sometimes, I just felt sorry for myself.

I finally got a boost in my energy when the cardiac medication dosages were fine-tuned. After several months of dragging myself around, at last I felt almost back to normal. In the spring, I received an invitation to review research proposals for the California Breast Cancer Research Program, the largest state-funded breast cancer research program in the country. Once again, having a chance to be part of reviewing scientific research proposals lifted me up and helped me to regain perspective on my illness and gave me hope again that one day, treatment and prevention would be very different.

…Be ground. Be crumbled, so wildflowers will come up where you are. You've been stony for too many years. Try something different. Surrender.

- Rumi

Chapter 12

Hollin's daughter, Naomi Elise Bley, was born June 6, 2003, in the late morning. Watching my daughter give birth was the most emotional event of my life. She was an Amazon -- strong, powerful, and determined. I was so proud of her. My stepdaughter Laura was Hollin's labor coach, and I got to cut Naomi's umbilical cord. She was long-legged and beautiful, with a head of dark hair.

Within 36 hours, my father passed away in Maryland, after years of struggle with dementia caused by a series of small strokes. We had life's major milestones as bookends.

Summer was busy with the aftermath of Naomi's birth and Daddy's death, plus the increasing demands of my work. Hollin had the growing support of a strong friendship with a co-worker Rodney, that was deepening into love. They became engaged by summer's end.

My energy had been somewhat better as we adjusted my cardiac medicines, but as autumn came, I was dogged by persistent fatigue. In early September, I traveled to San Diego for a breast cancer conference sponsored by the California Breast Cancer Research Program. Three days after returning from California, I headed to DC to review once again for the DoD. I was pushing hard the week before I left for California to be able to leave my work in good shape and to get my reviews for the DoD finished and posted on the Internet review site, since the deadline would occur while I was en route back from California.

For several days before leaving for DC, we all watched the weather and our emails. Hurricane Isabel was roaring toward the East Coast and the Army had to decide whether to hold our review sessions, asking everyone to fly toward the hurricane. These were the last sessions of the fiscal year and about $60,000,000 in research money was at stake. They decided to go on with the reviews, but to try to get us out of Washington early, working the review panels on an extended schedule.

We met in Alexandria and the sessions went well. The hotel kept us up to date on local conditions and emergency procedures. We conducted our review sessions thoughtfully and with heightened efficiency, finishing by the earlier deadline set by the DoD. The skies blackened, the wind picked up, and the rain started.

A few reviewers got away before transportation shut down, but many of us got socked in by the storm. Hurricane Isabel had hammered North Carolina and Virginia but had lost some steam as she moved inland. She was still formidable but was now a tropical storm, packing lots of wind and the promise of flooding. Soon airports closed and trains stopped running.

The hotel regularly distributed instructions and updates under the doors of our rooms. We were told to keep the curtains closed and stay away from the windows. If winds became dangerously strong, we could take shelter in our bathrooms or in the interior conference rooms without windows on the first floor of the hotel.

Alone in my hotel room, with the Weather Channel running constantly in the background, I felt a sense of disquiet. I realized that it was unrelated to the storm. I lay still on the bed and checked in with myself, with my mind, my spirit, and my body. I felt that something was wrong. I reached up and ran my hands over my chest. I could feel a hard place over my sternum, tender to the touch. It's back, I thought with grim certitude. I didn't feel much fear. I felt more resigned to the relentlessness of this disease. I wasn't eager to share this news with anyone. I just needed to be with it for a while. I already had an appointment with Dr. Johnson in a few weeks. I knew that in the whole scheme of things, a few more weeks weren't going to make much difference at this stage.

The next day, the storm had moved on, petering out. Parts of Alexandria were flooded. The airports were not yet open. I was flying out of Reagan National, and its runways were still under water. Baltimore Washington International was closed because of power outages.

Midday, the airport was due to open a runway or two. I got a shuttle to Reagan and joined the hundreds of others in line to re-book our tickets. The tarmac outside looked desolate. There were very few planes at any gates. Pilots and crew were deadheading their way back to DC. It would take a while to get aircraft and flight crew to the airport to begin putting people on flights. I settled in for a long wait.

For a few weeks, I had been stirred by the desire to write letters to Naomi. At the time that this wish took shape, I didn't have a sense that my breast cancer was back. I was thinking about my overall health and wanting her to know me and to know my love for her. There were lessons and family history I wanted to be sure were imparted to her.

I remembered my own Grandmother Lang, who had died of breast cancer before I was even two. She is just a pretty photograph to me, her dark curls piled high over piercing eyes. My half-sister Audrey, who is 13 years older than I am, had sent me copies a few years before of letters that my grandmother had written to her when I was a baby. I was surprised and touched to see references to me and to how I pleased her as her new grandbaby. I mattered to her! I want to be deliberate about the things I will leave for my grandchildren, whether sooner or later. The letters to Naomi were born out of that impulse. In the airport, I found a shop with lots of different journals. I bought one, settled in on a bench facing the runways, and began writing the first of a series of letters to her.

Back home, my October 8 appointment with Dr. Johnson arrived. I sat Steve down before we went and told him, "I've got a place on my chest that is worrisome. I'm pretty sure that the cancer is back again." He looked scared but tried to reassure me. We went together to the doctor's.

I saw Dr. Johnson at 3:15. I showed him the place and joked with him a little. "Dr. Johnson," I said, "I know that I can be a real crock, worrying about every little cough or ache. You've learned to tolerate my pushiness and my need to be in the middle of my treatment decisions." He smiled knowingly, in agreement. "What I know about myself is that when it has been something serious in the past, I get real quiet inside. It's that way now. I really think that the cancer is back."

By 3:55, Dr. Johnson had arranged for me to meet my old pathologist friend, Sanford Sharp. He did a needle biopsy and by 4:05 came back into the room. "I'm afraid it isn't good news."

"It's OK, Sandy," I said. "I really already knew." He left the room and returned with Steve and talked to us both briefly together, saying that he'd have Dr. Johnson call us at home in about an hour. When Dr. Johnson called, he said that the next steps were the full array of scans: MRI's to supplement a CT scan I had a few weeks before (which had not shown anything) and, for the first time, a PET scan. We agreed that a multidisciplinary team conference was in order. It was scheduled for October 21. He also prepared me for the possibility of thoracic surgery, a prospect that shook me up.

The hardest part for me was having to tell those that I loved and who loved me that the cancer was back again. It hurt to see how scared and concerned everyone was. Hollin was also furious, at science I think, incredulous that all we had done over the years still hadn't killed breast cancer off. Steve was angry that I was going to have to go through treatment (and all that accompanied it) again.

While I could move to a frantic place if I thought about work and how to handle it, when I separated out the breast cancer itself, I found myself mostly calm. I felt a kind of surrender that I had never experienced before.

Green Card

A fundamental shift
    subducts inside me
    as I hear the news once again
    that my breast cancer has returned.
I know this negotiation so well
    yet find myself at the bargaining table
    without words of arbitration
    without demands from my side any more.
I am the British up against Gandhi.
I cede the flag.
I don't feel beaten
    but rather gently overtaken
    by what is true:

cancer is now a persistent, insistent part of me
and I cannot deny a part of myself
nor treat it as the enemy any longer.
I still want to live – sometimes desperately –
but we must peacefully coexist.
These rogue cells have been the occupying troops for ten years.
They are marrying local girls
and everyone has applied for a Green Card.

The center leads to love.
Soul opens to creation core.
Hold on to your particular pain.
That too can take you to God.

- Rumi

Chapter 13

There is never a convenient time to get cancer. In my case in terms of my professional life, there could not have been a worse time to have this recurrence. I was grateful that the weekend before I was diagnosed with the recurrence, I had finally been able to sit the exam for my professional credentials as a Certified Fundraising Executive. Back at the agency, I was about to offer a newly created marketing position in my department to a talented young man. As a member agency, we had recently received the go-ahead from our local United Way to proceed with a capital campaign beginning at the end of November, just weeks away, with a goal of $2,000,000. I had recruited the new marketing person to free me up to give my full attention and time to the campaign. Now I was facing possible chest surgery, definitely more treatment, and an as-yet-undetermined amount of breast cancer. Again, the scans would tell the tale.

I felt both dispirited and amazed that this cancer had been so good at getting around all of the standard treatments we had slammed it with so far. It had recurred right in the midst of where I had been thoroughly barbecued with radiation two and a half years before. It had also recurred once more while on what doctors considered an effective oral breast cancer medicine. Puzzling over this with me, one of my friends said, "There must have been three cells left, and boy, were they pissed!"

The prospect of thoracic surgery still had me agitated. The scheduler from radiology calling and uttering the words, "The MRI of your chest and *brain* is set for Friday," was also a little chilling. But, generally, I was awake, aware, and mostly peaceful. I did talk once more with my oncologist about my fears and questions about thoracic surgery. I pictured the ventilators, chest tubes, and days in the ICU that I knew would be part of the immediate post-op time. I wondered about what they could do with my sternum. After all, the sternum is a key part of the skeleton, a linchpin. If I had to have my sternum removed, wouldn't my bones just fall in a heap to my ankles? He said that reconstruction of the sternum is possible – big surgery, but possible. While my number one fear was metastases to major organs, big thoracic surgery ran a close second.

Once again, my boss could not have been more supportive or flexible. I arranged my hours to accommodate all of the diagnostic tests I needed to have. We called in the young man to whom we had offered the marketing position and laid out the whole situation for him, right down to the worst-case scenario. He still took the position, much to my relief and delight, and he did the lion's share of the essential grunt work of the campaign over the subsequent months. I guided and directed but we would have derailed without his tireless detail work. He kept the wheels on the tracks.

October 21 finally arrived. Steve and I met with my treatment team and reviewed the results of recent tests, as well as the plan for what would happen next. The good news was that my lungs and brain were clear. The doctors took time to take us up to the lighted screen and point out areas on each scan. Next the thoracic surgeon spoke, saying that he was not enthusiastic about a surgical intervention. He weighed the potential long-term benefits against the complexity of the surgery, the chance of infection, the diminished function caused by moving abdominal muscles up into the chest, the problem with the area healing since I'd had radiation there. It didn't take long to cross that off the list. The bottom line for the thoracic guy was that if in exchange for such radical surgery he could be certain that he had gotten all of the cancer, he might be more in favor of doing it. Since the cancer was already throughout my chest muscle, it was unlikely that he could get it all.

I felt a huge sense of relief at having thoracic surgery eliminated from the treatment possibilities.

After a little bit of a scare with a spot that looked like it was on my liver, further tests ruled that out. The doctors concluded that this was a further extension of my last recurrence.

Next, my medical oncologist would decide what chemotherapy to use. We agreed that if I could qualify for a Phase II clinical trial, this might be the time to look for one. He would take a week or two to research opportunities and see if I met the criteria of any current trials. I was concerned that if I kept going through the ever-shortening list of chemotherapy available to me, I might eliminate myself from a clinical trial that could be helpful to me. Despite his extensive investigation on my behalf, I did not qualify for any Phase II trials that were available either locally or at larger centers like Vanderbilt, University of Alabama at Birmingham, Johns Hopkins, Duke, or M.D. Anderson Cancer Center in Houston.

The pathologist, Dr. Sharp, had done further tests on the tissue sample from my most recent biopsy, and found that it was HER2 positive. Evidence of this gene mutation represented a change and an unexpected finding, given the kind of cancer I have. We were dealing with a probable subset of tumor cells that were more aggressive. The good news was that there was a specific genetic therapy, Herceptin, which I could take intravenously to block the effects of the protein over-expressed because of this gene defect.

Dr. Johnson also decided to put me on Xeloda, an oral chemotherapy agent. This drug would be metabolized into 5-FU, like the IV chemo I had taken back in 1994. Xeloda was used widely in recurrent breast cancer. Taking an oral drug sounds like it should be easy, but I found myself surprisingly reluctant to take it as I stood at my bathroom sink the first morning with the pills in my hand. This took a conscious effort, knowing that it would likely make me feel lousy. I realized that letting someone else give me IV chemo was much easier for me.

Xeloda was fairly caustic for me. I had a full-blown toxicity reaction to my first dose, which made subsequent rounds of it, even at lesser dosage levels, hard for me. I was miserable for the first six weeks. I didn't eat any solid food from Thanksgiving until December 17 and became the cream soup connoisseur. The doctor kept ratcheting the dose down, but I became progressively more and more reactive to it.

After several rounds of the drug, Dr. Johnson decided that my body's hypersensitive response to the Xeloda was beginning to outweigh the potential benefits of the drug. My feet were so fiery red and cracked that I was unable to wear shoes. I scuffed around my office in overstuffed teddy bear slippers that a friend had given me, grateful for the padding that kept a cushion between me and objects I might bump with my feet. I had lost toenails, and the cuticles on both my hands and feet were inflamed and painful. Cancer can surely be humbling. It has challenged any sense of vanity I might have had.

I would never have imagined that part of my beauty routine would involve veterinary products. Although I coated my hands and feet often with Bag Balm, a lanolin-based salve used to heal dairy cows of cracking and chapping of their udders, no amount of moisturizing seemed to be able to keep the skin from getting worse and worse. I had ulcerations on every mucous membrane surface in my body, from stem to stern. I had long since given up wearing my contacts, plagued with running eyes and a dripping nose 24/7. A friend of mine from my therapy group named Deb, who also took Xeloda, laughed hysterically with me later at a little complimentary kit provided by the pharmaceutical company for patients about to take Xeloda. It contained a tube of Udderly Smooth Udder Cream (another popular brand among cows) in anticipation, we supposed, of the almost inevitable hand/foot syndrome. There was an entertaining little video about Xeloda therapy, just in case you didn't have anything interesting from Blockbuster to while away your evening. Finally, there was a little information card, with a profile of a red human figure seated on a commode, the person rendered in the international style as depicted on traffic signs. "Look!" Deb crowed, throwing us into spasms of hysterical laughter again. "It's the universal sign for diarrhea!"

In spite of the uncomfortable side effects, we could actually see and feel the tumors shrinking. It made the misery of those months worthwhile. Dr. Johnson discontinued Xeloda finally toward the end of February, but I had plenty of time to reflect on the experience.

Xeloda

I find it excruciatingly hard
>*to place these capsules in my mouth*
>*and swallow.*
Perhaps it is a metaphor for learning
>*to swallow the reality*

of chronic breast cancer.
I am surprised at how much easier it was
to submit to IV chemo.
This oral ingestion, day after day,
in my own home,
Requires an act of will, not submission
Purposefully taking these peach-colored tablets
that I know will make me sick
while, hopefully, making me better.
Xeloda sears me --
Scalds me from the inside out,
Blasting me from the ground zero of my insides
To the fire-stormed perimeter of my outsides.
I've swallowed a nuclear warhead
and every day
I'm given the red button to push to detonate still another.
Yet, like the utter vaporization of a hydrogen bomb,
I am amazed to watch and feel
my breastbone tumors shrink and disappear,
leaving little craters
where once the mushroom cloud bloomed.

Off of Xeloda now, I find myself emerging
from the nuclear winter of its aftermath.
The persistence of life awes me
as the springtime arrives again
My skin new
my fingernails growing out again
But with marks like charred rings on a tree
showing where the fire swept through.

During those hard months of treatment from November 2003 through February 2004, I was sorting through the feelings about this latest recurrence and my relationship with the disease. I felt very anchored in the decision that I was going to live as long as I could with as much presence as I could muster and try not to waste a lot of energy and time on what I couldn't fix or have mastery over. I knew that I wasn't going to die in the next week. I was highly unlikely to die in the next six months or a year, and I could even live to a ripe old age. After watching my father die of dementia at almost 90, I had also learned that there are things a lot worse than cancer.

I recalled some lines a friend had quoted to me from the *Grumpy Old Men* movies in which Walter Matthau and Jack Lemmon's characters are reflecting on the recent death of a mutual friend. The conversation went something like this:

"Did you hear about Chuck?"
"No! What happened?"
"Massive heart attack. Took him right out."
"Lucky bastard."

Few of us get to die in our sleep with our full faculties intact at ninety-five. I was just grateful to have had nearly ten years that I might not have had. I had raised Hollin, done meaningful work, sung, traveled, written, been blessed with mature old friendships and the great gift of new friends. I had married my soul's partner and dearest companion during those years. I was hoping to live lots more years, but balanced with knowledge of the fact that none of us gets out of here alive. The guiding principle that I adopted was, "I'm not going to die every day until I die."

I began to think of breast cancer now not as an enemy and

not something to fight. Somehow, all the military comparisons and martial language that had helped me gather strength and determination to face my initial diagnosis and treatment just didn't seem appropriate any more. This "invader" was a part of me now. I wasn't giving up, but the path that I needed to take was now one toward peaceful coexistence with my cancer. I still prayed and hoped for its remission and quiescence, but breast cancer seemed to be a part of my interior landscape.

I still wanted healing, but I was beginning to understand the difference between healing and cure. It seemed that in order to get that healing for myself – spiritual, emotional, and hopefully physical – I needed to learn to accept this thing that I once regarded as alien as now a part of me.

After he discontinued the Xeloda, Dr. Johnson ordered scans again to see how I had responded to the treatments. I was preparing myself as best I could emotionally. I was ready for a little progression of the disease and would have been happy to hear that it was relatively stable or somewhat diminished. What I wasn't ready for was the news that there was no evidence of cancer anywhere on the PET scan. I was in full remission once more.

I mouthed the words to my rejoicing family and friends, but I felt like my emotions were not even in the neighborhood of what my lips were speaking. This notion of peaceful coexistence with breast cancer was sometimes an uneasy truce. I hit the wall about a week after I got the news.

P.O.W.

The good news shatters me:
There is no residual evidence of breast cancer –
for now.

Even my breastbone,

> *whose structure had been seized by those cells*
> *that hunkered down and claimed territory*
> *with stubborn squatters' rights –*

Even it is totally clear, abandoned by those tenants.
I am numb –

> *not elated or relieved.*

My head hears the words and registers them

> *at the highest cortical levels,*
> *that the threat is gone,*

But my reptile brain

> *skitters for the shelter of the shadows*

and my heart cannot trust to follow along at all.
A week later, life outwardly normal, I find myself sobbing

> *as I drive to work.*

I have a sudden image of myself

> *as a prisoner of war.*

I am taken, over and over again,

> *before a firing squad,*
> *awakened in the night*
> *or pulled away from my breakfast*
> *by my captors,*

Who tell me that the time has come.
They blindfold me

> *and lead me stumbling to that wall.*

I hear the gunmen assemble,

> *the click of their rifles*
> *as they check the ammunition*
> *and release the safety.*

I wait to hear the bullets' report,
wondering if I will die before or after the shots are audible.
Ready, aim, fire!

I brace for the onslaught
   but smell only lingering Cordite,
   not the silver scent of my own blood.

The soldiers have fired their guns in the air.

My knees buckle in a strange sense of betrayal,
the reality that I am about to die
   stripped from me once again.
Saved, but naked,
   I am blinking in the sunlight,
   left alone by that wall as the soldiers disperse
   in this odd, dependent dance with my captors,
   masters of fear and hope
   who still hold the keys.

I hear the jingle in their pockets.

*Today, like every other day, we wake up empty
and frightened. Don't open the door to the study
and begin reading. Take down a musical instrument.*

*Let the beauty we love be what we do.
There are hundreds of ways to kneel and kiss the ground.*

- Rumi

Chapter 14

Sometimes denial is a useful thing. During this time of re-mission, I decided that I would do my best to put breast cancer up on an imaginary shelf and live my life. I was still receiving the genetic therapy Herceptin weekly, but I had no side effects from it. I call it "chemo-lite." Herceptin and my daily oral dose of Aromasin were the gentle reminders that we were still patrolling the borders of my cancer, but there was nothing more intrusive than that. I had real life things to prepare for, like Hollin's wedding.

I slowly regained some energy during the spring of 2004 and really enjoyed the preparations for Hollin and Rodney's wed-ding, which took place on May 16. It was a beautiful day, and they were married in a glass pavilion adjacent to a park in downtown Chattanooga. They rode in a horse-drawn carriage to Chris's res-taurant for a lovely reception. Hollin was a gorgeous bride. Rod was so handsome in his tux. Little Naomi was irresistibly cute in a frothy white dress with lavender embroidered flowers and soft crinolines. It was a perfect day. Several times, I caught myself grinning and thinking, I'm alive to see this!

Steve and I got away for a few days of R and R the next week, to our favorite beach in Gulf Shores, Alabama, bordering the Florida panhandle. The stress of treatment, the stresses of work, and even the happy stress of planning and hosting a wedding had taken their toll. The beach is the quintessential healer for me, and we hardly left the beach except to replenish our seafood stores.

We also began looking forward to a family vacation in the Gulf Shores area in mid-July, with the whole Hampton clan, kids and grandkids. When I had first had a recurrence in 2000, I had made a wish list of things to do, to spur me on instead of continuing to postpone plans and to give me goals and things to look forward to. A family trip to the beach was high on that list. The recent return of the cancer had made the urgency of fulfilling that wish more alive for me, and the family was excited to plan the trip.

This time of peace and better health was short-lived. In mid-June, I found another lump on my chest and knew that the remission was over. Dr. Johnson ordered the usual battery of tests. In late June, we found out that not only did I have a 3-centimeter lump in my chest wall, I also had two lymph nodes in my chest, under the breastbone, that were showing cancer.

Steve was so angry and discouraged. He said, "There's no place to hide from this stuff."

I agreed and told him, "All we can do is to walk out to meet it." We didn't yet know how to do that, but we would learn as we went along.

I told Dr. Johnson about our family's planned trip to the Gulf and that I was not going to miss it, period. He agreed and said that depending upon the timing of my treatments, he could even find a way for me to get a treatment in Mobile (about 45 minutes from the beach), if we needed to.

The doctor began me on gemcitabine, another IV chemo-therapy that I would take in cycles of three weeks on, one week off. With each treatment, about six hours after the IV infusion, I experienced full-blown flu-like symptoms for about 48 hours: shaking chills, some fever, muscle aches, and a headache that lasted for five days. This drug also rapidly tanked my blood counts. First, my white counts dropped and, for the first time in all of my treatment history, I required a shot to stimulate the production of white blood cells. Second, my platelets dipped precipitously, not quite to the level where I needed a transfusion, but to 30,000 -- enough to make me darned careful when I was chopping onions! The weekly finger stick at my doctor's office took 15 minutes to stop bleeding. Finally, my red blood cells plummeted, producing anemia, with hemoglobin levels of 8.2, also requiring medicine to stimulate the production of new cells. I was dragging myself through the days.

The family trip to the beach became my touchstone, my reward to myself for getting through the treatments. Our mid-July vacation time finally came and my blood counts were low, so Dr. Johnson withheld treatment that week. Hollin, Rod, and Naomi were unable to come, but the other 11 of us happily inhabited a beautiful three-bedroom condo right on the Gulf of Mexico for a full week.

We played on the beach all day then enjoyed each other in the evenings. Our family loves to play all kinds of games: cards, board games, charades, word games – you name it. We're a rowdy, mouthy, competitive bunch. It's not unusual for the whole group to unite against someone if that person is winning a game by a mile. "Let's get him!" becomes the rallying cry.

We were playing Royal Casino, one of our favorite card games, and I was doing very well. We were six adults and a couple of grandkids around the table, and everyone began taking potshots at me, teasingly. Finally, Steve piped up, "Oh, sure! Gang up on the girl with cancer!" There was a collective gasp around the table, and then everyone just completely fell apart laughing. I laughed hardest of all. The energy released by that ironic joke was immense. For several weeks, my illness and the recent bad news had been like the proverbial elephant in the living room that everyone had been tiptoeing around. For the rest of the evening, I had a new nickname that everyone tried out, saying it out loud. "Cancer Girl" joined "Cabana Boy" and the other vacation-generated nicknames. It was great! It was recognition that this is part of what is normal in our family. We needed to be able to talk about it and yes, for God's sake, to joke about it sometimes, too.

I was so proud of my family and my husband. In one moment, they embraced what was true, named it, and defined it as part of the reality of our family. They trusted me and where I was with it enough to make a joke, to do the normal thing that they would do under any other circumstances. What a powerful model for our grandchildren about how to deal with life! That simple action opened the doors to much franker discussion than our kids thought they had permission to broach. It also set the stage for support and planning I would need later.

During this time, I revisited my relationship with my illness. I still felt committed to learning to live with this thing, but a friend called me to some balance about it. I had embraced metastatic breast cancer enough to feel some emotional peace, but a friend pointed out to me that I nearly always said "my breast cancer." She raised a good question: did I want to own it and accept it to that extent? Initially, I responded by saying that acceptance of it was essential to my mental health, but her question left me thinking about what messages I wanted to send to the cancer. How could I be a realist in order not to get yo-yo'ed around too much emotionally by its persistence and yet maintain awareness that this was a disease process and that I might have some say in mitigating its effects?

As sometimes happens in that state between waking and sleeping, I had a vivid dream. I pictured my body as a vast, lovely national forest. My chest wall was an area designated for campers – not as pristine as the surrounding forest, but maintained with still a semblance of the original woods, contained and monitored, with rules governing who stayed there and how they were to behave. The "campers" were the persistent chest wall lesions. I had a vision of the cancerous lymph nodes as some rebellious campers out in the virgin forest, lighting their campfires without any regard for the danger to their surroundings. I saw myself as the park ranger, confronting them and saying, "Hey, you yahoos! Whaddya think you're doing out here? You can't camp here! Put out that fire! Are you crazy? You could catch the whole woods on fire! You could burn this whole forest to the ground!" In the final scene, I firmly escorted them out of that area and reiterated the rules about the designated camping area.

It made an impression on me. I felt comfortable knowing that I could deal with this disease if it stayed somewhat contained. I did not, however, have to lie back and let it overtake me, at least not without some screaming and hollering at it. So, every morning, I called up that image and told the doofusses to put out that fire and get out of the woods!

The gemcitabine really kicked my fanny all summer long. Like when I was on the Xeloda, I became progressively more reactive to it, ending up with vasculitis (inflamed blood vessels) in my legs. Vasculitis in my legs could mean that other organs were at risk, like my kidneys. Dr. Johnson discontinued the drug. Despite all the misery, Dr. Johnson and I could both feel that some of the places on my chest were actually bigger. It was time for scans again.

I lay on the CT scanning table, trying to steel myself for the results. I knew that we would have to do some other kind of treatment, but at this point, there were only two conventional treatments left for me. We were definitely getting down to the short list. I had some larger questions to consider, too. Given how sick I had been throughout the summer, if the treatments left to me would keep me that sick, was the trade-off in my quality of life worth it? If I didn't take treatment, what kind of life would I have? Did I have the strength to go straight into rigorous treatment again?

Lost Summer

A lost summer,
> *that time compassed by chemotherapy*
> *viewed through the watered glass*
>> *of weariness*
>> *so bottomless*
That I cannot invoke any impression
> *of those days.*
Cancer in its cunning
> *has run all the roadblocks.*
The pockets of my hope
> *are turned inside out.*

Dr. Johnson reviewed the CT scan results with us. The news was not good. Despite Herceptin and gemcitabine, the cancer had progressed. One more lymph node in the chest was now affected and there were two nodules on the lining of my lungs. I asked Dr. Johnson about how ill I felt. Was it the cancer that was making me feel so terrible? He answered that my inflammatory response to gemcitabine was the worst that he had seen, and it was the drug that was making me feel awful. He reassured me that as I recovered from its side effects, I would begin to feel better.

I was so sick – sick physically and sick of cancer. I was utterly exhausted and, for the first time ever, feeling ill equipped to advocate for myself. I needed to take care of myself but felt that there was no way to without also working at my job. Steve was self-employed and I carried the health insurance for our family. But I just wanted some relief.

What I really longed to do was to stop working and to use this time to devote to my total health. That desire seemed completely out of reach as we stepped into a new phase of my treatment.

Dr. Johnson felt that it was time to investigate Phase I clinical trials at M.D. Anderson and at the San Antonio Cancer Institute. He would begin researching my eligibility and investigating what was available at those centers. He felt more confident about my chances of qualifying for a Phase I trial, in which drugs or combinations of drugs are tested for the first time in humans. Dr. Johnson offered us some reassurance that he was basing his optimism about my qualifying for a Phase I trial on the fact that I was still relatively well and strong. I was open to this and Steve was supportive.

I hated to see the fear and sadness in Steve and Hollin's eyes. I wished that I could take it away. I felt so helpless. Logic told me that my being sick was out of my control, but sometimes I felt that it was my fault that everyone was worried and sad. In thinking about my illness and myself, though, I felt mostly calm, perhaps pulled back from the fear, and occasionally angry that the cancer just kept marching on. Steve talked some, sharing his sadness and fear for me, for us, and for himself. He was extra tender with me, one night stroking my hair until I fell asleep.

Hollin woke me up one night, wanting to talk. She wanted to be sure that I wasn't sugarcoating any of the news that I was sharing with her. Finally, she wept and said that she wanted me to live long enough for Naomi to remember me. Then, in a small voice, she said, "I don't know what I'm going to do without my mama."

She touched me so deeply. We cried together. I told her that was a question that all of us face. We can't answer it until we live through it. I said to her how proud I was of her and how confident I felt that she would be fine and able to handle her life. I let her know what a wonderful young woman I saw her becoming. I was so glad that she had said those hard-to-say words. Once again, as much as I hated being sick, cancer was the matrix for deepening my relationships, pushing me and those around me to get down to the real stuff.

This new set of clinical findings upped the ante for me. For well over a year, the theme of so much of my journaling and reflection had been trying to gain balance in my life. I wanted to reduce the stress levels, pare down my calendar and level of busy-ness, and lighten the material load at home. We had created an apartment in our downstairs for Hollin, Rod and the baby, remodeling the area into 1500 square feet of living space with a full kitchen and their own private entrance. In doing this, we had already had to lose half a house in possessions. It had felt wonderful to jettison things and begin to simplify. Now I felt even more urgency about getting things done.

Where could we go from here?

Within a week of talking to Dr. Johnson about Phase I clinical trials, he had found that there was nothing at that time at M.D. Anderson for me, but there was a study in San Antonio for which I had a high probability of qualifying. Six days after our discussion with Dr. Johnson, Steve and I were on a plane to San Antonio for an appointment at its Cancer Institute. I was half-excited and half-anxious to see what they might be able to offer me and what it would require of me. I feared that if I qualified for a trial I might have to live in Texas for its duration, away from my family. I could see myself in some generic furnished apartment, with motel furniture, lying in bed alone, wandering from room to room, looking forward to personal contact with my doctors or nurses at whatever happened to be my next medical appointment. If that was a requirement, I didn't think I could do it. My emotional reserves were so low.

We arrived in San Antonio the day before my appointment. The end-of-August heat took our breaths away. We took a shuttle from the airport to our hotel, one of those recommended by the Cancer Institute offering a special rate for their patients. We found ourselves on the outskirts of town in an area of apartments, strip malls, and medical buildings. Steve decided that we needed to rent a car so that we could go back downtown and get a feel for the city.

We spent our first day in San Antonio enjoying their River Walk, a beautiful respite from the summer heat. We ate great Tex-Mex food and ambled along the river. We were aware how weighted each moment was with our hopes and fears. Truthfully, we were running low on hope.

Later that evening, we stopped for coffee at a restaurant on the River Walk, and Steve asked the strolling mariachi band to play me something romantic. "Loco," a song about being helplessly in love, became the background music of our time in Texas.

I fell into restless sleep that night, knowing that the next day would significantly shape my life, our lives.

The next morning, we drove to the Cancer Therapy Research Center (CTRC), which, in collaboration with the University of Texas Health Sciences Center, comprises the San Antonio Cancer Institute. The CTRC provides the largest Phase I clinical trial program in the country. We entered the Grossman Building, feeling somewhat desperate. What if I didn't qualify for some trial here? My treatment options were becoming so limited. We hoped that the doctor could offer us something – anything – that might be a reasonable match for where I was in my disease.

Many of the patients in the waiting room reflected the population we had seen in San Antonio the day before, largely Latino. I thought how wonderful it was that such a great resource was available for people locally or within a reasonable drive of San Antonio. At the hotel, we had already met other cancer patients from around the country. One man from Florida with advanced renal cancer was doing very well eight months into his trial, with his tumors receding. That's the kind of news I wanted to hear!

The nurse called my name and Steve and I went back to the exam room, awaiting our meeting with Dr. Quincy Chu. We pictured an austere, serious researcher. I expected a reserved and formal Asian-American and hoped that he would be responsive to our anxiety and questions.

Dr. Chu swept into the room, a ball of energy. He exploded any worries I had that I might need to pump him for information or be concerned that he might be aloof from us. He was expressive, talkative, bright, appealing, and funny. He rapidly gained our confidence and engaged us both intellectually and emotionally. He had reviewed my history thoroughly and felt that he had a study that would be a good match. He reassured us, saying that my cancer was still comparatively slow growing, even though it was resistant to the recent treatments I had been taking. He reiterated Dr. Johnson's assessment that I was strong and relatively well and therefore a good candidate. He explained the hypothesis behind the proposed drug combination he would be using, watching us carefully to be sure that we understood the science behind the study. He neither talked down to us nor talked over our heads.

The drugs were oral and taken daily. I would need to travel to San Antonio more frequently initially to have blood studies drawn. Once that was completed, my visits would be monthly, for a checkup and to get the next month's supply of the experimental drug. I would take the experimental drug, GW572016, in combination with an approved estrogen blocker called Femara. GW572016 had been tested in many other solid tumors, alone and with other proven therapies. This study was the first pairing with Femara, and I was one of the last two patients to enroll worldwide in the study. He told us some promising preliminary findings of response to this combination, even in very aggressive breast cancers.

The side effects would be a nuisance but seemed manageable. The most common were diarrhea and an acne-like rash. I knew that as a test subject in a clinical trial, I would receive first-rate care and careful monitoring.

Dr. Chu stressed the importance not only of my understanding the informed consent documents but of Steve, as caregiver, being completely familiar with the drugs and possible side effects, too. He sent us off for the rest of the day to talk over participating in the trial and to review thoroughly the consent forms, making an appointment to follow up with us the next morning. His research assistant, Missy, met with us, too, and explained the consent portion. She became a great resource and support for us.

We left the CTRC early in the afternoon. The time with Dr. Chu altered my perception of how treatable I was at this stage of breast cancer. Both Steve and I felt hopeful and uplifted for the first time in months. We returned to the hotel and rested for a little while, aware of how taut our nerves had been and how limp we now felt from sheer relief. Late in the afternoon, Steve suggested that we drive downtown again and enjoy walking along the river.

We stayed down at the River Walk until late that evening, eating various courses of our dinner at different restaurants. Every time Steve saw a mariachi band, he would ask them to play "Loco," tipping them generously, expansive with happiness. We were both high on hope.

I placed one foot on the wide plain
of death, and some grand
immensity sounded on the emptiness.

I have felt nothing ever
like the wild wonder of that moment.

- Rumi

Chapter 15

On the practical side, we had to figure out travel money and time. The drug company supplied the medication used in the clinical trial and covered any medical expenses not billable to insurance, but travel expenses were ours. Our cheapest airfares by far were through Southwest Airlines, flying out of Nashville. That meant that a trip to San Antonio took a minimum of three days, with a travel day on each side of the appointment day. Steve insisted on coming with me. I felt that I could do it myself after this first time, but he recognized how weakened I was from the gemcitabine chemo I had taken all summer. Looking back, I realize how frail I was after nearly a year of chemo and the side effects of gemcitabine.

During this difficult financial challenge, we received help from unexpected sources. Sometimes anonymously, sometimes directly, friends and acquaintances stepped forward and assisted with our travel expenses. This was the beginning of a humbling time. Over the next months, we learned to accept love at a new level and to allow people to fulfill their impulse and desire to be of some help.

Working out the time off at my job was difficult. My boss and our Board Chair were extremely supportive and flexible, but I was rapidly coming to the end of all earned leave time. I was more and more aware that the demands of treatment were elbowing their way in front of the other responsibilities in my life. Thankfully, our capital campaign was moving toward successful completion of the $2,000,000 goal. The dilemma about what to do about work took on greater and greater importance.

Between the end of August and mid-November, we traveled to San Antonio seven times. Steve always accompanied me. After trying to walk the long concourses in the airports and having to stop and rest repeatedly, I finally relented and let Steve ferry me through the airports in a wheelchair. A side benefit was that using a wheelchair also gave me preferential boarding rights, which was essential. On the GW572016, my intestinal tract became unpredictable. It was crucial for me (and for the other passengers) that I could be seated near the restroom on the planes and that I could be among the first off.

We spent two of our trips to San Antonio doing the special blood studies that the clinical trial required. This portion of the trial is called "pharmacokinetics." It measures the activity of the drugs at very specific times after taking them. I had to stay in the treatment room of the CTRC for most of the day, with blood being drawn every 15 minutes, then every half hour, then every hour, the intervals becoming increasingly spaced out over 12 hours. This is a critical part of the research. The nurses set a timer to signal when the next sample of blood was to be drawn. In a room of 30 patients receiving treatment, probably half of us were doing the pharmacokinetics element of our trials, so the room was filled almost all the time with the crazy cacophony of cooking timer beepers going off.

I was so grateful for Steve's presence. I was touched as I watched him creating his own glossary of cancer terms. During the pharmacokinetics visits, tears sprang to my eyes as I saw him, head down, concentrating on carefully copying the times that the nurses were to draw my blood. What a life for him... He has always been an active partner in my care and in whatever I faced.

Crate

My love,
How different this deal has turned out for you.
While not a new car on the lot of your life,
    you chose me,
    a dependable classic
    with some zing under the hood.
A vintage GTO, perhaps,
    a little bit jazzy
A convertible
    with new chrome rims
    some engine modifications
    a soft interior
    and a new paint job
Nearly restoring me to my former glory;
Even some funky fur dice
    hanging from the mirror.
Once you drove me off the lot, however,
I began dollaring you to death
    and I know that I wasn't what you had bargained for,
    maybe a car built on a Monday.
The engine rebuild came without a warranty
    and soon I was limping along
    with little power or responsiveness,
    the ragtop dry-rotted by age and deteriorating

and the paint job, just an Earl Scheib special.
Even the dice are now a moth-eaten,
        sun-faded gray and white.
Yet, miraculously,
        you don't act as though you've been cheated.
You take me out often.
You even visit the dealer regularly
        and shake his hand.
You pat my peeling paint affectionately
        and look at the sun through the holes in the roof.
You putter down blue highways with me,
        choosing to watch the scenery,
        eschewing the freeways and the speeds
        that I no longer can sustain.
Amazingly loyal,
        attached to this wreck,
        still able to see its beauty,
Committed to the journey.

The name of the game with cancer is adjust, adjust, adjust. The side effects of the clinical trial arrived as predicted, which provided an ironic feeling of relief in me. After my unusual reactions to Xeloda and gemcitabine, predictable was good. In addition to a GI tract that functioned at warp speed, I had gotten the lovely acne, too, on my face and even into my scalp. Fatigue was a persistent feature, too, although we didn't know if this was mostly the drug or the wear and tear of travel. I just settled into it as "normal."

The clinical trial required a CT scan every two months. I had one in September, as I began the study, and November brought the next one. I was able to have the CT's done in Chattanooga and would then take the reports and all my films with me to my appointments in San Antonio. Before our trips to San Antonio, I would pick up the radiologist's report and films myself, so that I could hand-carry them to Dr. Chu. I could choose whether to read the results on my own in the parking lot of the imaging center. Cocooned within my purple PT Cruiser, I couldn't resist. Not knowing made me more anxious than reading the results on my own.

In mid-November, I picked up my scan results on the Friday before we were due to fly to San Antonio on Monday. I sat in my car and pulled out the report. The CT showed "significant progression" of the cancer in the chest wall, with one sizable tumor mass pressing up against the brachiocephalic vein, a large blood vessel that is an important route from the arm and the head back to the vena cava, the major vessel that empties directly into the heart. I had been experiencing some pain in my left shoulder and along the left side of my neck, as well as in my chest if I stretched my arms out. This new development explained it.

I knew that this degree of progression meant that I would have to come off the study. I was eager to talk with Dr. Johnson about the CT report but missed his call on Friday. On Sunday, Y-ME had a big fashion show and fund-raiser. Hollin and I were among the models for the fashion show, and Steve and other friends and family were in the audience. Dr. Johnson was one of several doctors who had agreed to be escorts for the models. When he saw me, he offered to stay after the event and talk to me about my CT results. I had the films and reports in my car, since we were getting ourselves together for our trip to San Antonio the following morning.

After the fashion show, Dr. Johnson sat down with Steve and me and generously gave us about a half hour of his time. He was very concerned about the progression of my disease. The clinical trial had stabilized some of the lung lesions, but this progression in the chest wall was apparently serious. Dr. Johnson was trying to be gentle with us in introducing the bad news. When I asked about the chest wall mass pressing up against the brachiocephalic vein, in an endearing, avoidant moment of medical double-speak, Dr. Johnson said, "We could be looking at a life-limiting event."

Well, if that wasn't some do-si-do and allemande left around the hard truth! The combination of anxiety and absurdity made me burst out laughing. "You mean that it could kill me, don't you?" I asked, bluntly.

"Yes," he said, softly.

I got my emotions in check enough to be rational about the next part of our discussion. Dr. Johnson was kicking into high gear on my behalf while we were out of town. He would schedule a PET scan and MRI for the day after I returned and a multidisciplinary team conference as soon after that as scans could be read. He told us that he wanted the thoracic surgeon present again at the consultation to revisit whether chest surgery was necessary or advisable at this point to deal with the threat of the chest mass. He was so kind and concerned, and we were very grateful that he gave us so much of himself and his time on his day off. I was so tired and disheartened I just wanted to lay my head down on the table among the discarded napkins and cutlery, close my eyes, and escape this new set of facts.

We traveled to San Antonio, each of us quieter than usual, alone with our own thoughts and concerns, arriving on Monday afternoon. I had a heart scan scheduled for early Tuesday morning and would see the doctor early Wednesday. After the scan early on Tuesday, we drove out into the Texas Hill Country to pass the day and take our minds off the worries about my health.

We saw Dr. Chu on Wednesday and he formally took me off the study. We told him that at this time, we wanted to consult with my health team back in Chattanooga about conventional treatment and to hear what their advice was about the latest findings. He reassured us that there would always be Phase I opportunities for me, should I ever want to come back for another clinical trial. I had received excellent care in a truly patient-centered environment. Although the experimental drug didn't work for me, I later read that it was effective in about half of the breast cancer patients treated with it. I was glad to have been part of the study and to have added my share of data to the scientific findings.

I spent the next day, Thursday, back in Chattanooga going from one test to another. Friday morning, Steve and I were to meet again with the treatment team. I was scared about what the scans had shown and about what the doctors would recommend. The prospect of thoracic surgery loomed large in my mind once again.

We met with the treatment team and they presented a plan. The scans showed lung and liver involvement, multiple lymph nodes in my chest and left armpit, and chest wall tumors. Rob Headrick, the thoracic surgeon, and my general surgeon, Laura Witherspoon, talked about thoracic surgery again, ruling it out. Since I now had well-established organ involvement, and considering the same concerns as before about healing and disability after surgery, operating on my chest wall and sternum did not provide benefits that outweighed problems. Dr. Witherspoon expressed her belief that had we done thoracic surgery a year ago, it would not have gained us anything. "I firmly believe that we would be sitting here looking at the same scan results, and you would have had a miserable year," she concluded. Dr. Headrick nodded. Steve had been second-guessing the decision from the year before about not pursuing thoracic surgery. I was relieved that he could now let go of that concern.

The immediate treatment goal was to shrink the chest wall tumor that was pressing on the brachiocephalic vein. This area was giving me substantial pain and I was back on narcotics to get relief. Dr. Kimsey, my radiation oncologist, spoke next, saying that the treatment team agreed that the highest priority was to begin radiation therapy as soon as possible. He also ordered a bone scan as a baseline, since it had been a year since I had one. It revealed cancer in my left collarbone, too.

Dr. Johnson spoke next, saying that as soon as the radiation therapy was over, he would do a CT again and then begin chemo-therapy with Taxol and carboplatin, three weeks on and one week off. He also said that other treatment options for me included going back on Xeloda at a lower dose and taking it continuously, moving on to Navelbine (which I had never taken), or considering using Alimta, a drug used in an aggressive lung cancer that should be approved any day for use in metastatic breast cancer.

Although I was feeling overwhelmed, I was also awed to think that in August we had two treatment options but we now had four. I reminded myself that my work was to stay alive and relatively strong long enough for the next treatment to come down the chute. In just three months, new choices had become available.

The doctors – my friends – around the conference table asked me where I was with all of this. I said that I was just so tired, so tired. I expressed aloud my wish that I could stop working and take this time for myself, especially given the grimmer outlook for my prognosis now that I had several organs involved.

Laura Witherspoon looked at me and said, "It sounds to me like you've already decided to stop working. Now your job is to figure out how to do it." That one statement enabled me to embrace the possibility and finally to move to make it happen.

As Steve and I left the conference room, I knew that I was about to step on the treatment merry-go-round once again, and it would be going 90 miles per hour. I was going to have to concentrate on willing myself to jump on, grab it and hold on once again. It seemed so long since I just had some relief.

That afternoon, I was in Dr. Kimsey's office, stretched out on a table, with my upper torso held still in a hard foam block, as he did my radiation therapy planning with the CT scanner. Having my arms over my head and lying motionless hurt my chest so much. The pain was a mix of burn and ache. By the end of the 45 minutes that it took him to define the treatment fields and plan his approach with a CT machine, I had tears running into my ears.

I began radiation therapy right before Thanksgiving and finished a few days before Christmas. As treatment progressed, the pain in my chest wall lessened. This time, I did not get a radiation burn, just a new permanently tanned area on my already colorful chest. I had an annoying cough by the end of treatment, but did not have the very sore throat that might have happened as a normal response. My most vivid memory of this time is hearing the same Johnny Mathis Christmas CD every single day as I went in for treatment. It may have ruined Johnny Mathis for me forever.

Facing the new serious level of concern about my long-term health (read: "longevity"), lots of change was in the wind. As we shared the discouraging news of the spread of the cancer, people began responding. I began to get phone calls, letters, and emails from concerned and caring friends and family, offering every possible alternative medical approach. This was a little touchy. One thing I've learned for myself and in working with other women with breast cancer is that you have to make the best possible treatment decisions for yourself. The ideal is to make an informed decision that will help you feel as whole as possible, will allow you the degree of control that is comfortable to you, and will help you not look back later and regret or second-guess your decisions. Those decisions are as individual as each woman is.

When friends offered me information on treatment, especially if it was an alternative to conventional therapy, I thanked them and reviewed it with an open mind. The therapies people offered included everything from Chinese medicine to vitamin therapies to special diets and herbal remedies to enemas, and then some.

I knew women who drank wheat grass infusions. I knew women who took what back in my days as a nurse we used to call "Three H Enemas" --high, hot and a hell of a lot. All of these therapies have their proponents and testimonials about success. At this stage in my disease, I didn't want to overlook any opportunity, but I also needed to be realistic with myself about my high degree of comfort with conventional medical treatment.

I did not choose at that time to pursue any of the alternative methods of therapy, but I did begin to explore complementary approaches. I began using the services of my hospital's Cancer Resource Center, enjoying massage and Reiki, a practice that originated in Japan, which uses what Reiki practitioners call "life energy." It produces deep relaxation and some people report healing.

Being a conventional science person, I had what I call "healthy skepticism" about Reiki. I met the licensed clinical social worker, Gerre Schwert, who was a trained Reiki practitioner. She had worked at Yale in its bone marrow transplant unit and had received training from the Center for Mind/Body Medicine in Washington, DC. We talked about this modality for me. It would consist of a half hour or so of sustained light touch to areas of the body that reportedly were channels for life energy. I figured, what could it hurt?

The first time that I had a Reiki session, I was surprised and impressed. Using my reference of Western science, I don't understand how Reiki works, but I can't deny what I experienced. I lay on my back on a massage table and first Gerre held my head, changing position three different times. Her hands were cool as she did this. Next, she laid her hands lightly on my collarbones and chest. Within seconds, I felt as though she had placed a heating pad there. It was amazing. As she moved to the other sites on my hips and knees and then my feet, her hands remained warm and my body felt warm. I sank into a deeply relaxed state, my limbs feeling very heavy. I've tried to continue with a Reiki session every week.

Gerre also helped me with deep breathing and some basic meditation techniques. This has been a good resource for me in periodic and systematic relaxation. She has also become a friend and sounding board as I've worked through issues about death and dying. In combination with my therapy group of women with advanced breast cancer, I'm well fortified.

When the news of my more serious disease was shared within our family and among our closest friends, I had several people step forward, wanting to talk frankly and openly with me about what I needed and how they could help. My oldest friends Betty and Dorothy and my stepdaughter Laura were particularly present in dealing with the possibility of my dying sooner rather than later.

Betty and Laura asked me to go out to dinner with them. We had a wonderful, open, frank conversation about my worries and concerns, the things that I wanted help with right away and the things that I want to be sure would be tended to after I die. I talked about who I needed to write my obituary, and the need to pull together a box with materials to meet the religious requirements of our faith for burial. I talked about my wishes for my memorial service and where my email distribution list was, so that friends could know when I was either too ill to write them or when I died. I asked Laura to help her father with the details of insurance, taxes, and those things that he hates to deal with and isn't particularly savvy about. We laughed and cried, and these two sweet souls helped me to focus on issues that I felt I had been carrying mostly alone. Steve was just not ready to look my death in the eye yet. Hollin was still young and consumed by the responsibilities of work and her family. Laura and Betty were the perfect people to walk with me toward this possibility and to share the load.

During this time in late 2004 and early 2005, I also looked for

ways to direct my writing and thinking toward end-of-life prepara-
tion. There are plenty of resources for people experiencing grief after the loss of someone they love, but there is very little out there for
the person going through this experience. I realize that once most
of us have dealt with these things, we die before we can reflect on
what was useful or write a "how to" book for those who follow us.
I found a few books that were helpful and began using them as a
study guide. The real work, however, was in plain, old-fashioned
soul-searching.

Dance, when you're broken open.
Dance, if you've torn the bandage off.
Dance in the middle of the fighting.
Dance in your blood.
Dance, when you're perfectly free.

- Rumi

Chapter 16

When I was first diagnosed with breast cancer, I felt such desperation and terror. The fierce drive I felt to live to raise Hollin to adulthood powered much of that feeling. I had mourned the things I thought I would not get to experience or see. For one thing, I had wanted to hold my grandchild in my arms. I had that longing fulfilled with the wonderful grandchildren Steve brought me through his children and then by watching Hollin give birth and become an incredible mother to Naomi. I also had the icing on the cake of my loving extended family.

I became more and more aware of the net of prayer that was woven around me. Since the first days of my initial cancer diagnosis ten years before, I had so many people offering prayers on my behalf. During this time, I felt that support increase exponentially. People called or emailed me or greeted me at the mall or at the hospital with the words, "We're praying for you!" Sometimes I didn't even know these people; perhaps they were a friend of a friend of a friend. Every Sunday in our worship service, I was remembered by name in the prayers of my own Baha'i community. Chris and Jen hosted a prayer breakfast for me one morning that was so powerful and moving as family and friends gathered and prayed for me and with me. My own prayer was to lean into God's will, whatever that was to be, and for strength and trust in the ultimate goodness of that.

I realized that I was at a stage in my life and in my illness where I saw that this world and life after death were more of a continuum rather than an abrupt change or division. With each recurrence, I had stepped closer and closer to the fact that I am going to die eventually. The tests that cancer brought me had challenged and finally deepened my faith. I believe with absolute certitude that this life and its difficulties are for our spiritual development. The hard stuff burnishes our spirits. My soul is my reality and the part of me that will have existence beyond here. I found comfort and ease in that knowledge. I had given up trying to puzzle out the fairness or unfairness of cancer. There was always the tension, however, of that certitude, and my breast cancer as a physical presence and weight that I was pulling around with me. Sometimes I just wanted to be free of it, but I knew that just the act of struggling to haul the truth of my cancer around with me was transforming. I had watched so many friends live with courage and die with grace. I felt that I had the tools I needed to approach my own death as a transition and as another opportunity for growth and intimacy with those I love.

An interesting outgrowth of this reflection was that while I still felt like a separate species sometimes, just as strongly I was aware of my connection to everyone and everything around me. That awareness brought sweetness to every day.

The winter of early 2005 was a time of both practical and introspective end-of-life work. I was able to do this because I decided to stop working. It was a very hard decision, and I knew that it would create a financial strain immediately. We had blown through

$10,000 of savings in medical costs in less than five months. I was beginning to have to draw money out of my IRA. Despite that, I just couldn't marshal the energy to continue work. Beginning in mid-December, I started my 90 days of medical leave to which I was entitled under the Family and Medical Leave Act. I had used up every hour of my earned leave time, both vacation and sick leave. Those 90 days of unpaid leave would meet the requirement for consideration for long-term disability benefits provided by my agency. I would also apply for Social Security Disability.

My friends and co-workers hosted a luncheon for me that last day. It was bittersweet. Everyone knew the sub-text: Debbi isn't likely to return. It was a loving gathering of well-wishers with everyone's homemade goodies. My friend Ken Clay even theatrically rolled a cart of fresh ingredients right up to where I sat in the place of honor and prepared a huge bowl of his killer guacamole, which I relished.

Having worked nearly all of my adult life, I was concerned that I might become depressed or feel bored without the structure of work each day and the presence of a community of co-workers and friends. That wasn't the case. For one thing, as I began little by little to undertake work around my home, I became fully aware of the cost of my illness over the past five years in chaos and disorder. I had worked full-time and that had been about all I could manage. Being home gave me the chance to reclaim my household, to rest and nap when I needed to, to go to lunch with friends and renew friendships that I had neglected for lack of time and energy.

I soon found that I needed to fine-tune how I structured my own time. It was easy to be passive. Early in my days at home, I spent a whole day in my pajamas and watched the TLC channel on cable from 9 a.m. until 9 p.m. Whoa! I pulled myself up short at the end of that day and said, "Your brain has been massaged to mush by hours of the perfect proposal, the perfect makeover, the perfect remodel, the perfect wedding and the perfect birth. You'd better limit TV and be sure that you get dressed early in the day, every day." I decided to restrict my TV viewing to no more than an hour and a half a day. Soon, medical appointments and treatment demands gave plenty of structure to my calendar and to my days anyway.

Before I began my chemotherapy of Taxol and carboplatin, I got to try out my oncology office's new CT scanner. I've had at least a dozen CT scans over the years and the machine cues you when to breathe, usually in terse American phrases: "Take a deep breath." "Hold your breath." "Breathe." Dr. Johnson's office bought this brand-spankin' new machine from Siemens and apparently, the English-speaking option was British English. The first time I was in the machine, the vocal cues were, "Take a deep breath." "Hold it right there!" and -- the pièce de résistance --"Carry on breathing!" I was laughing so hard I was quivering. They had to start the whole scan over. I told the tech that they needed to create a redneck prompt for us Tennesseans: "Suck in a big one!" "Awright now, hang onto it." "OK, let 'er go."

The baseline scan showed the same thing it had six weeks before: lymph node involvement inside the chest, lung lesions, a small liver lesion, chest wall involvement, and a lymph node under my left armpit. The area where I had been irradiated showed the tumor as smaller. I began my treatment with Taxol and carboplatin as the year turned to 2005.

One of the paradoxical and peculiar things about cancer for me is that what is at times dramatic eventually becomes, at some level, ordinary. The experience of treatment, the contemplation of my mortality, the occasions of receiving and absorbing calamitous news over and over again, are profound and also curiously mundane. Catastrophe becomes commonplace. I don't mean to diminish the seriousness or importance of these events in my life (especially as fodder for change and growth), but I have found that I can only sustain for a limited time this sense of medical melodrama that has characterized so much of my life over the past 12 years. At some point, it all seeks its own level and becomes routine, with the patina of disaster dulled by repeated exposure.

By the time that I began my chemotherapy at the beginning of 2005, a year of constantly doing one kind of treatment or another had made this newest regimen just one more thing to be done. The challenge in entering this new treatment was that I was totally exhausted. My white blood counts rapidly dropped on the first round of treatment. I began getting Neupogen shots four or five days a week to keep those numbers up and enable me to get all three treatments in each cycle. My life was totally medicalized. Now in addition to my accustomed weekly trips to the oncologist's office, some weeks I had to be at the hospital six days out of seven.

After a few weeks of treatment, I began to experience shortness of breath on the least exertion. I wasn't anemic and I didn't have pneumonia. Dr. Johnson ordered a chest X-ray and we were surprised to see that half of my diaphragm was paralyzed. We still don't know definitively why this happened. I also saw my cardiologist and he ruled out any more dire reasons for shortness of breath, including inflammation of the lining of my heart and any possible clots on my lungs. Further evaluation showed that my breathing wasn't compromised enough to require oxygen, just enough to be uncomfortable. One more adjustment! One interesting and welcome side benefit of all of this diagnostic work-up was that in mid-February, the CT of my chest ordered by the cardiologist to rule out blood clots in the lungs showed that the tumors were significantly smaller. The chemo looked like it was working already!

I spent the winter and early spring in 2005 working my way through items on my "get-your-life-in-order" list. I revisited my estate planning and revised terms of my will. I formalized my list of tasks to delegate against the time that I wouldn't be able to do things for myself by virtue of illness or my death. Steve remained standoffish about these issues, changing the subject or quickly reassuring me that I would be fine. I didn't want to push him too hard, but I was concerned that there were things that we needed to talk about, that he needed to know about. Other than being present at my lawyer's office to review the changes in my will, he did not want to talk about any of the specific things that made the possibility of my death seem real.

Steve had persistent bronchitis in late January and February. He coughed up some blood during that illness and his internist referred him back to his pulmonary doctor. That doctor said, "Steve, it's probably just the force of your coughing that has produced blood, but with your history of smoking, I have to look further." Steve had quit smoking the previous summer, but we knew that he was still at higher risk for lung cancer. The doctor ordered a CT scan, which was normal, but he felt that he needed to do a bronchoscopy. What if he had lung cancer? I had visions of us sitting side by side in the treatment room, each hooked up to chemotherapy, playing cribbage until one of us literally pegged out.

Steve has a terrible fear of choking. He was very anxious about the bronchoscopy, more from that fear than worry that he might have cancer. I walked into the computer room at home the night before his procedure and found him typing. "What are you working on?" I asked him.

"You need to know where these things are," he answered. "I've written letters to you and to each of the kids and grandchildren. If something happens to me..."

"Do you feel intuitively that something is going to go wrong?" I asked.

"I'm just so scared of choking to death," he answered.

I hugged him and tried to reassure him that the procedure itself would maintain an open airway by way of the scope. After a few minutes, he showed me where on the computer to find the file with the letters. This was my chance.

"Honey, while we're looking around the computer files, let me show you some things, too." I leaned over his shoulder and opened files and documents of my own, with instructions and information about what to do when I die. We both held each other and cried but it felt great to get all of that out there. Steve's own realization that something could happen to him opened him to understanding my need to share my arrangements and provisions, too. I finally felt connected to him around these crucial issues. The door was open to talking about the hard stuff and I was determined to keep my foot firmly in the doorway.

Steve came through the brochoscopy without any problems and the findings were negative for cancer.

I settled into the routine of getting the Taxol and carboplatin. My hair fell out early into the treatment. I wore my old wig for a while, but it was pretty worn. Handling and exposure to heat while cooking had made it look ragged and frizzy in places. Even the skills of the man I had bought it from couldn't completely restore it to being presentable.

I had a chance to tag along with some long-time girlfriends, Lois and Mary K., on a trip to New Orleans in April. We stayed at the home of Lois's sister. We had so much fun enjoying great food, art, shopping, and time together. On one of our shopping forays, Mary K. reminded me that she had offered to buy me a new wig for my birthday, the previous month. We stopped in "Fifi Malone's" in the French Quarter and she bought me a wig in a sleek pageboy. If I combed it just right, I could burst into a Streisand medley without much provocation! It felt so much prettier than my old ratty wig.

Cumulatively, taking the chemo was beginning to knock me down. I was having more nausea after each treatment, but could push it back with Zofran. I was more tired than I could ever remember. Afternoon naps became a regular part of my days. I was pale and drawn, and my hairlessness accentuated how sick I looked. Also, for the first time, I was completely devoid of body hair. Eyebrows, eyelashes and every other place were naked. I felt disempowered by this, as though my status as a grown-up woman was compromised.

The month of May brought a welcome relief from all the medical things that were running most of my life. Hollin, Rodney, Naomi, Steve, and I went to Gulf Shores for a week in mid-May. Some dear friends gave us a week at a hotel there for some real relaxation and family time. Watching little Naomi revel in the beach and the ocean was a joy, day after day. The weather was gorgeous, and I came back feeling rested, with some much-needed color to my skin. All of this took place during a hiatus of three weeks in my treatment, so I felt the best I had felt in over a year. I was quite a sight on the beach in my two-piece. I cut a lovely figure at my weight of 166 pounds, more than I weighed at nine months pregnant. I was anemic and pale as a fish belly, with layers of radiation tan all over my chest and those pretty little spider veins that come afterwards. I had no boob on the right, my port-a-cath sticking up through my skin on the left, no eyebrows or eyelashes, yucky Taxol toenails -- ahhhhh, Cancer Girl was back on the Redneck Riviera and still standing!

Wearing the wig was so hot in summery weather. It felt like having a plastic grocery bag on my head. Rivers of sweat ran down my face. About halfway through the week, I ditched the wig, moussing down my three-quarters-of-an-inch-long silver-white hair. I just finally thought, I'm still here, by God, and I'm going to relax and quit worrying about how I look.

When I returned to Chattanooga, the weather was warming up there and I decided to go without the wig. My stepson, Chris, said that I looked like I should be in a James Bond movie. You know the type of female character: "The sex was great, Mr. Bond, but now I'm going to have to kill you."

In late May, Dr. Johnson did a CT scan, to see where things were at this stage of treatment. I was hoping that I might be able to take a complete break from chemo for a while. The scan showed that the lung and liver lesions were clear, but there was still evidence of cancer in lymph nodes in my chest. We needed to keep on with the treatment.

One day, after being on Taxol and carboplatin for more than six moths, I suddenly had a major allergic reaction to the carboplatin. The Taxol is usually more likely to elicit an allergic response, but this time it was the carboplatin. About ten minutes into the carboplatin infusion, I suddenly got hot, itchy, and breathless. Apparently, my face was cherry-red. My lips started tingling, as did my hands and feet. I suddenly felt just awful. I spoke up quickly, saying, "Hey, something's really wrong with me." My chemo nurses are excellent, and they were on top of what was going on immediately. They got a doctor into the treatment room, pushed more Benadryl on me, gave me epinephrine, started oxygen, and nursed me through the GI symptoms that developed quickly.

The event was oddly reassuring to me. As this incident rapidly developed into a full-blown anaphylactic reaction, I felt myself pulling inward. I wish that I could say that my life flashed before my eyes or that I had some profound revelation. To be honest, what I thought was, Oh, hell! I never got the cars re-titled in both our names!

I felt the room around me recede. Sound was softer. I could feel Steve holding my hand and I was aware of lots of activity around me, but I felt like I was in the middle of a lake, floating. All the activity was happening on a distant shore, on my periphery. I thought to myself, Well, this could be it. I might be dying. I didn't feel scared at all. I felt peaceful and unconcerned, detached from all that was happening outside of myself. I actually remember little else of that whole afternoon. The nurses got me stabilized and sent me home. I took Benadryl around the clock for two days, sleeping most of the time.

That experience really reduced the fears that I had about the process of dying. I still feel scared sometimes about what physical challenges might lie ahead – pain, dependence, loss of bodily functions – but going through that episode reassured me about moving through death itself.

Through the early months of summer, I continued on the Taxol alone. Finally, it was time to scan again, this time with both a CT and a PET scan. Dr. Johnson was out of town so we set a date for the first day that he was due back to review the results. I used to want to know the results of every test immediately. I have gotten to the point where I think that bad news can keep. Whatever is already is.

PET Scan

The increased metabolism of cancer
    lights up a PET scan
    like city lights
    or the spangled nightscape
    of networked airport runways.
I lie here under the scanner
    wondering how months
    of carboplatin and Taxol have affected my cancer.
Don't let me be O'Hare
    and the distant sparkle of Chicago.
I want to be the Badlands of South Dakota

Bleak

Godforsaken

and blessedly black on the screen.

Steve and I sat waiting for Dr. Johnson. He came in and sat down, as he had done so many times before, and we waited to hear the news that would determine how we would live our lives for the next months.

"Lungs, liver and all those lymph nodes in your chest and armpit are completely negative right now," he said. "Everything is completely clear, except one little place on your chest wall."

The three of us grinned at each other. Another reprieve.

Life is ending? God gives another.
Admit the finite. Praise the infinite.
Love is a spring. Submerge.
Every separate drop, a new life.

- Rumi

Chapter 17

Breast cancer has been like a foreign country that I've had to learn to live in. When I was first diagnosed, it was as though I had been parachuted into enemy territory, an unwilling draftee, and I had little knowledge of the terrain. I had to learn the language and customs of this new place and learn them quickly, as though my life depended upon it -- and it did. I had to understand its culture rapidly and make decisions in a hostile environment, decisions that would affect the rest of my life and that might determine how long I would live and what my life might be like.

I found myself homesick. I wondered if I would ever be able to go home again. I missed my old life so much and just wanted it back. I knew that I was engaged in a war that was going to change me forever, but I had no idea how profound that change was going to be or where it would take me. As the years went by, the war was over but there was no going back. This new country became my permanent assignment and then, truly, my home. My memories, my accomplishments, my ties are built on this land.

After 12 years, I have now spent one third of my adult life in this place. Its hills and valleys have become as familiar to me as the recollections of my childhood home, so far away. I did not choose this place as my homeland but it chose me. Each experience, each encounter has harrowed up the soil of my life, my heart, my soul. In that well-tilled soil, I have set down roots and have seen the fruits come up. From this ground, I have learned of my capacity for courage, acceptance, strength, humor, joy, and persistence. I have come to know and trust myself.

I have a friend who has been quadriplegic since he was 16 years old. When I first got to know him, I was in my late 20's and he was in his early 30's. In the first days of our friendship, we talked about life and where we were at that early stage of our adulthood. He spoke about his physical limitations and his adjustment to becoming paralyzed at such a young age. I remember that I was amazed (and perhaps a little dubious) to hear him say that if he could do his life over to that point, he wouldn't change the fact that he experienced an injury that caused him paralysis. He was fully aware and remarkably grateful for what such a test and challenge had brought to him, how it had affected his very soul, and to the good.

My illness has brought me its own tutorial. Looking at where I am now, at the changes that breast cancer has offered and forced in my life, I understand my friend's certitude in saying that he wouldn't change his life. For as hard as this has been, I wouldn't change my life. Breast cancer has been a huge test and a blessing. If I weigh it all out on my own scales of understanding, the blessings side is far heavier.

Breast cancer has been a tough teacher, but it seems that the demanding instructors are the ones we remember as the best ones. This teacher has expected much of me and calls me to learn lessons and step into territory that I didn't know I could even attempt, let alone begin to master. The common thread in this education of my heart and soul has been about living with breast cancer, not dying from it.

One aspect of this schooling has been my relationship with myself, both my physical self and the core reality of my self. There has been an ebb and flow in my relationship with my body. I have always enjoyed being a girl. I don't remember ever once wishing that I were a boy. I was well into my thirties, however, before I began to enjoy paying attention to my looks and finding my own sense of style. By age forty, I felt competent in this area and confident about how I presented myself. Breast cancer challenged me on every front. When I first had cancer, the loss of my breast wasn't important in the face of my fear that I could lose my life. When I had the second mastectomy, I realized how breasts had been a hallmark of my being a woman and even of looking immediately recognizably human. Deciding later upon reconstruction brought me to a new phase of my relationship with my physical self. Then losing my reconstruction because of recurrence and the body changes resulting from nearly constant treatment over five years has made me confront and revise my view of my physical being many times.

My relationship with my physical self now is sometimes uneasy and ambiguous. I thank this body of mine that has rallied and responded to treatment so many times, that has shown strength and endurance in the face of a persistent assailant. Yet I sometimes still feel betrayed by it, too. Why does the cancer come back and come back? I see my many scars as evidence of a series of battles, sometimes as signs of having been violated by this disease, but more often as badges of effort and even courage.

We live in a society that defines our worth and identity by the images of advertising and by the calibration of material measures. Are we thin enough? Tall enough? Pretty enough? Youthful enough? I've been forced to try to let go of those assessments and to concentrate on my internal reality. After all, if I live long enough, aging will finish what cancer has started for me in stripping me of the "marketable" measures of beauty. Maybe I'm lucky to have a head start. This physical framework is so transitory in the grand scheme of things. I'm not saintly at all about this. I have to discipline myself to pry my fingers from my attachment to how I wish I still looked and felt physically. But I remember that profound truth that imbedded itself in me years ago and cling even harder to it: it's how I live my life that matters.

I try to keep my focus on knowing that my worth and that of everyone I encounter lies in the fact that we are all a reflection of God's image. It's plenty enough work in whatever remains of my lifetime to develop those godly attributes latent in me of mercy, kindness, peace, justice, and so many others. It's plenty enough work and delight to use this time to try to build community and relationships that foster the emergence of those qualities in others.

I have spent these years with cancer looking for its higher purpose in my life. I don't profess to have some cosmic understanding of that, but every day I see evidence of the gifts that it gives me and the opportunities it opens to me. I think that when we suffer, we have two choices: we can become involuted, bitter and blaming, or we can dredge out a deep channel for compassion and see ourselves linked to the suffering and struggle of other people.

I try to make thankfulness central to my life and to each day. It's really not that hard. It can even become a habit. It takes an open eye and a willingness to frame each hour in wonderment. I love how the morning sun's slant is beginning to change as summer ebbs. From my porch, I laugh at how the red-bellied woodpecker scares himself as he swoops in and lands hard on our bird feeder, then seems to look around to see if anyone noticed his awkward touchdown. I listen to my youngest grandchildren playing, the sound of their laughter sweet with its own music. Each week in the chemotherapy room, I am struck speechless by the kindness shown among the patients, the sick reaching out to others who are sicker or more fearful, reminding me that people are essentially so good. There are the small pleasures of each day, too. I can call up how my daughter's hair smells, wet and clean after a shower, how a freshly unfurled newspaper feels like vellum, or how the bed lightly creaks as my husband turns in his sleep and reaches toward me.

Few things pass me by now. I'm so grateful for this mindfulness.

Living with the uncertainty of my life is sometimes still trying. When I'm sick from the cancer, the urgency is high to continue working on getting my life in order and dealing with end-of-life issues; but the problem is that when I don't feel well, it's hard to muster the energy to get on with it. When I'm feeling well and have the energy, the heat is turned down on the urgency. The end-of-life work that I've done this past year as my prognosis worsened has been helpful, necessary, and meaningful. Now that I'm doing better, though, sometimes I feel like I'm all dressed up with no place to go!

I can get grandiose and think that I know that it's breast cancer that will be the cause of my death. It seems that when I'm in that place, something happens that reminds me how none of us knows what our own end will be, and I certainly don't. One time, I was in a car with my boss, and a logging truck that had lost its brakes blew through a traffic light and missed hitting us by inches. Another time, I was hemmed in at a traffic light and a car was hurtling toward me in the wrong lane. At the last possible second, the car almost supernaturally veered through bushes into the parking lot of a fast food restaurant, becoming airborne and then jolting to a stop. No one was hurt and I didn't die, which had seemed inevitable as I watched that car bearing down on me. I guess I need dramatic reminders that I'm neither omniscient nor omnipotent. It's good for me to be humbled.

Sometimes, my world (which seems so normal to me) collides with how the majority of the world lives. I was walking with a girlfriend a few weeks ago, and we were talking about home projects. She and her husband live on the beautiful lake that spreads out behind TVA's Chickamauga Dam. She was getting estimates for having their boat dock rebuilt after flood damage and general wear-and-tear. As we walked in the thick morning air of late summer, she said, "I really liked the contractor I just met with yesterday. He understood how to stage the project so that we could do one portion now and another portion next summer and another portion the summer after that."

My knees nearly collapsed as my reality smacked up against hers. Planning for two summers down the road! What an amazing concept! I was both awed and amused to think about how, in my world, the four months that Dr. Johnson estimated until he would do another scan on me feels so long – luxuriously long. It represents the largest time span I've faced in over two years without a doctor expecting to peek into me to see what's going on. Looking ahead two summers? It's just not in my repertoire any more. I don't envy my friend her point of reference for time and planning. I'm just aware at times like these of how fundamentally different my own life is.

So, the trick seems to be walking the tightrope between maintaining hope that I could live to a ripe old age and living for and in this moment. How can I feed my hope? I do it not by focusing on the physical and material aspects of my illness but rather by focusing on the other things I envision in my life. If I focus on my breast cancer and my physical history of recurrence, I wouldn't feel very hopeful at all about my life. My spiritual and emotional history, however, tell me that I have every reason to be filled with hope. Where my hope lies is in my sureness that I will be able to face whatever comes and that I won't have to face it alone. I'll have within me and around me what I need for the journey, wherever it takes me.

Having watched a number of friends who have died of breast cancer, I know the unpredictability of my illness at this stage. I have had friends to whom I've spoken and who seemed stable, and four weeks later were gone. I've had other friends who I thought could not possibly live out the year, yet who are still managing. I run into them at Target, as they shop for yet another season of school supplies for their kids. That seems to be the nature of metastatic breast cancer: the course is not always predictable, and it's rarely a straight-downward nosedive.

I feel like a leaf in the wind. I'm hedging my bets that breast cancer will be what takes me out, but I don't know for sure. By now, I know the steps of this dance, but sometimes the music changes unexpectedly. Right now, I'm riding the updrafts for as long as I can.

Some people talk about cure, but I don't have that word in my personal vocabulary, at least not where it applies to my life. I've watched other women live out their lives meaningfully, right up to their deaths. Were they cured? No, not if you mean having their illness taken from them and living on without breast cancer. Were they healed? By my witness of their lives, yes, they were healed. Their lives were as whole and authentic and full as any I've ever known, whether they lived to be 28 or 80. That's the healing that I pray for. Make me a whole person, one who loves and accepts and serves and rejoices and opens myself to others honestly and without hesitation.

Then I might be someone worth remembering. Then I will have left a life well-lived.

Surrender

My surrender
>> is not a weak-kneed act
>> but a genuflection
>> a gesture of homage to all that has happened,

The blood and the blessings,
>> each pass of the knife
>> a cleansing stroke

Until my heart lay cleft,
>> and surrender became deliverance
>> renunciation.

I am unburdened
>> bird-boned
>> traveling Light
>> ready to fly.

Appendices

An Informal Guide for Dealing with Issues Related to Metastatic Breast Cancer

Facing Recurrence and Uncertainty

When I had my first recurrence six years after my initial diagnosis, I was so angry. I had done everything that I could the first time around to be aggressive in attacking the breast cancer: bilateral mastectomies, chemo even when it wasn't strongly recommended, Tamoxifen... Yet, here it was back again. It took me several months just to sit with the anger until I worked my way through to several realizations. First, I could reassure myself that I really had done everything possible the first time around and I just happened to be one of those who fell on the wrong side of the probability statistics. Second, I saw that while I didn't have control over anything about this disease, what I did have control over was how I responded to it. From that time on, I began to learn to live with the uncertainty that comes with metastatic breast cancer. I have been through several more recurrences since that first one and now am in treatment all the time, but managing it.

For me, when the first recurrence happened, I felt like the scariest thing I had feared had happened. The amazing thing was that even that was survivable. Facing metastatic disease has its own challenges and scares, but the one fear of recurrence that had loomed so large in my mind had occurred, and my world is still going on, five years later.

At this stage in my disease, this is not a battle any more. All of the military language of fighting cancer just is not as comfortable for me now. When I was first diagnosed, I really did need to marshal all my forces, emotional and physical, to try to obliterate my breast cancer completely. What is more useful for me now is learning to coexist peacefully with breast cancer. After 12 years, this is part of me. Breast cancer has been with me one third of my adult life. Like any other chronic disease, it's something that I have to accept and work with. That's not to say I'm giving up or that I don't want to live. I have so much to live for and so many things I want to do. I can spend my energies better not railing against something that is so unpredictable. I try to look for the lessons breast cancer has to teach me.

Dealing with metastatic disease involves adjusting and readjusting your expectations, hopes, and what you regard as normal, over and over again. When the cancer spread to my lungs and liver, we hung onto the "good news" that there was only one lesion on the liver, less than a centimeter in size, and that the lung lesions were just on the lining of the lung.

Remission is a wonderful thing, but I'm also a realist. I've been in and out of remission several times, so the path across that threshold is getting well-worn. I'll ride out the times of remission for as long as they last. The name of the game seems to be "Stay

Well Enough until Something New Comes Along." The wonderful news is that each year, there are new therapy options. A year ago, I had two conventional, approved drug choices left to me. Now I have four, so it's not over yet.

The uncertainty is difficult, but I try not to dwell on it. Early in my disease, when a holiday or other special milestone came along, in the back of my mind would be a little voice saying, "This might be the last time…" Recurrence has helped me to flip my perspective around and each milestone has become a cause for celebration. "Wow! Another wedding anniversary and here I am enjoying it!" I try to stay in the here-and-now.

Family and Children

With the diagnosis of metastatic breast cancer, spouses, partners and children have to face a new reality, too. They have to face an increased likelihood that you'll die of this disease. They have to give up their wish that everything would just return to and stay "normal." Just like we have gone through periods where, more than anything, we just want our old lives back, they go through that, too, perhaps even more when there is recurrence.

It's important to keep the lines of communication as open as possible. At this stage, it's easy and tempting to begin to protect each other from hard truths and scary possibilities. If this happens, it begins to make distance between you and your spouse or you and your children, at the very time when all of you need extra closeness. Some family members will just not be able to deal with this degree of "bad news." Find your support where you can. With immediate family, it may take your initiating and raising things that concern you or need to be taken care of. In the case of my husband, I'll confess that I shoved on him from time to time until he was willing to hear me out on issues I needed to discuss, from revising my will to my wishes about how I want to be cared for. I've been blessed with children who are very frank, and that is a relief to me. My daughter always wants to know exactly what is going on. My stepson calls often just to check on how I'm doing after a treatment or test.

When I had news of my lung and liver mets, my stepdaughter immediately asked to meet and talk with me. We talked, we cried, and we planned. She was concerned about how her dad was handling my illness and prognosis and how he would handle my death. She and a dear friend of mine sat down with me and said, "What things are you most worried about that need to be taken care of now and later?" We made a list together and assigned people to deal with things that I worried about, things that I wouldn't be able to take care of if I were too sick or things to take care of after I die. What a burden was lifted from me by their willingness to be so open to me and with me!

Support from other Women with Stage IV Breast Cancer

Even with excellent communication with family and friends, there is no substitute for talking with other women who are dealing with similar circumstances. Y-ME National Breast Cancer Organization has a 24/7 hotline (1-800-221-2141) that will hook you up to someone who understands and can relate firsthand to your feelings. You can call in the middle of the night, if you need to, when troubling thoughts or worries keep you awake and you just can't turn off your head and go back to sleep. Y-ME can even match you with a trained peer counselor whose course of illness has been similar to yours.

Locally, if you haven't participated in a breast cancer support group, this may be the time to do it. Beyond support groups, I have been so fortunate to have access to an actual therapy group for women with advanced breast cancer that our local Y-ME affiliate sponsors, co-led by two licensed clinical social workers. For me, talking with other women with advanced disease has been the best resource.

I believe that those of us with metastatic breast cancer need an arena in which we aren't editing ourselves to protect other newly diagnosed women. When I was first diagnosed, I wanted to see the women who were 10, 15, 20 years out and doing great. Women with recurrence scared me. I wanted to be done with cancer. I remember that feeling. At this point in my disease, if I meet a newly diagnosed woman, unless she asks me point blank if I've had recurrence, I just say that it's been 12 years since I was diagnosed. If she does want to discuss my recurrence, I try to reassure her that the vast majority of women do just great after treatment and that I'm an anomaly.

You may find a new friendship in the treatment room, talking with other women who are going through chemo for recurrence. I really do value the chance to talk without any abridging with other women who are ready and willing to discuss their experience with advanced disease.

Sexuality

Sexuality is one of the most neglected issues in cancer care, and especially in breast cancer. Because most of us have tumors that are estrogen-receptor positive, as soon as we are diagnosed there is an immediate impact on us biochemically as we get treatment that either blocks estrogen or affects our fertility and hormone balance. Combine that with changes in body image, chemo fatigue, all the effects of treatment, stress over work, finances, children... It's no wonder that we might have some difficulty in the bedroom! This is also the one area about which so many doctors get squirmy or want to pass the buck. "You really need to talk to your gynecologist," say many oncologists. "Maybe you really need to see an endocrinologist," say some gynecologists. Then the endocrinologists defer back to the oncologists, "I really couldn't do anything that might interfere with your cancer treatment."

In the meantime, you're trying just to remember what it was like to feel that wonderful warm tingle of desire. I found myself feeling like my aging had been compressed into just a few months, with changes in desire, response, and the physical changes associated with no estrogen.

Again, communication and talk about expectations seems to be so crucial. In my marriage, this has been an area of great adjustment. Before my recurrences, we had enjoyed a very free and rich intimate life in our marriage. Being in and out of treatment with chemo, radiation, and additional surgeries has definitely affected us. Changes in my physical appearance have also sometimes affected my confidence, and feeling sexy is rooted in confidence. My husband has been patient and incredibly affirming. He honestly still believes that I am the most desirable thing on two legs! We get lots of touching as part of our daily contact, even if intercourse does not happen with anywhere near the frequency it once did. We cuddle a lot and snuggle when sleeping, and we know that physical contact like that reinforces the bond. When I feel well enough, we make love. Sexual expression is still an important way to communicate for us, but we've both had to adjust our expectations and remain flexible in how we show our love to one another.

My internist (a woman) referred me to a wonderful gynecologist (a woman) who works with a psychiatrist (a woman) specializing in menopausal issues. Between the two of them, they were able to help me tease out what issues were physiologic and what were emotional responses to the stresses of having advanced breast cancer. The psychiatrist brought not only her understanding of human emotions to our work together, but also her knowledge of anatomy, physiology, and biochemistry as a physician. She has been an invaluable resource in helping me look at some alternatives.

Depending upon your temperament and openness, one thing that can be helpful is the variety of marital aids available now through other women who are selling accessories that can be incorporated into your intimate life. In the past, you might have had to go to some unsavory store on the sleazy side of town to see what's available, but not any more. This is an area that you and your spouse or partner might want to explore. I believe that these items are also available through on-line purchase, but I prefer to deal directly with someone I know and trust who is offering products through an established company. This was a "brave new world" for this 50-something woman, but it's been helpful for me and for us as a couple.

Depression and Anxiety

Dealing with the long-term uncertainty of metastatic disease can take its toll. Sustained stress affects your brain chemistry and can lead to depression and/or anxiety that may improve through medication and therapy. Don't expect yourself just to "tough it out." Facing this stage of my life is probably one of the most challenging things I've had to do and anti-depressants and availing myself of a good therapist have been a lifeline. If your partner or children are open to counseling, it can be helpful for them individually or with you, as well.

Clinical Trials

If you haven't yet considered a clinical trial, this might be a good time to discuss it with your oncologist. When I had just two or three treatment options left, we first explored Phase 2 trials, but I had difficulty qualifying. Several months later, we explored my eligibility for a Phase 1 trial and I qualified. I participated for several months out of state in a clinical trial and it was a good experience. I was monitored extremely closely, got excellent care, and felt that not only might this trial help me, but I was helping to advance research by participating. In my case, my disease progressed despite the trial, but I would choose to do it again. The research center where I participated also let me know that I should still consider myself as a probable candidate for other Phase 1 trials in the future, if I were ever interested again. They told me that for Phase 1 trials with breast cancer patients, they expect that we will have been through multiple therapies so the exclusion criteria are generally not as tight as for Phase 2 trials. It's still my "ace-in-the-hole."

Many larger medical centers are also satellite sites for clinical trials that are occurring at larger research facilities and universities. You may not have to travel at all or perhaps not very far to participate. It's worth investigating.

To Work or Not to Work

Throughout my breast cancer, it had been important to me to work. First, there was the simple economic necessity. Second, I was the one who carried the family's health insurance, since my husband owns his own business. Mostly, though, I enjoyed my work, and maintaining the structure of work and having something meaningful to do each day was vital to my sense of well-being and normalcy. I took very little time off for chemo and even showed up for work in sloppy tee shirts for a few weeks when I was trying to heal a big radiation burn. This wasn't heroic – it was for my mental health as much as anything.

This past year, I began to shift in my view of work. After 10 years of breast cancer, I was just plain exhausted. I calculated one time that if I included the time I was just on Tamoxifen or Arimidex, over a ten-year period, there had only been a total of five months that I wasn't taking some kind of treatment for breast cancer.

When I was dealing with my second and third recurrence and my treatment was virtually ongoing, I began to think about stopping work. When I had liver and lung mets appear, I took stock again about how I was spending my time and my life and what I still wanted to do, as well as what I had the stamina still to do.

I worked in a job with a lot of responsibility and multiple projects going on all the time. It was stimulating and very satisfying and I had a lot of opportunity for autonomy and professional growth. During the last year of working, I noticed some "slippage" in my memory and ability to concentrate. I began to worry that the time would come that my performance and the outcome of my work would begin to show the deficits I was beginning to feel. My boss and co-workers were extremely flexible and supportive, but the time came when I felt I needed first to take all the medical leave that was due me under the Family and Medical Leave Act and then to consider whether it was time to go on long-term disability. My increased absences to accommodate treatment requirements compounded my feeling that it was time to stop working, if I possibly could.

I took my 90 days of medical leave and, during that time, applied for my long-term disability benefits through work and through Social Security. I had used up my paid sick leave and the 90 days of unpaid medical leave were difficult financially, but I did qualify for disability after the 90 days and I retired officially at the end of my medical leave time.

It's a decision that I have not regretted for a moment. I had worked a lot of this through in my head and heart for about a year before stopping work, so I was ready. I thought that I might become depressed without the structure to my time that full-time work provided. This has not been the case for me. The demands of my treatment and my energy level benefit from not having to work. I have taken this time to do some of the things that I had put off. My days are full and I can rest when I need to. This is finally the time to take care of me. Some people take it when they are first diagnosed. For me, this is the right time.

Disability, COBRA, etc.

I have several friends with advanced breast cancer who found stopping work very difficult emotionally. To them, it felt like giving up and giving in. For one friend, this meant that she never completed her 90 consecutive days of leave in order to qualify for her employment disability benefits. It was hard financially as she became sicker and finally passed away. The disability income could have relieved some of the stress she and her husband were experiencing. I do, however, absolutely honor her need and desire to work for as long as possible. For her, it was part of maintaining her dignity and sense of herself. These are highly individual choices and are tied to issues of identity and self-esteem, as well as to finances.

When you are diagnosed with advanced disease, it's important to review your benefits and your financial situation. In my case, maintaining my family health coverage was crucial. It's costing me about one third of my monthly disability income (and my disability income is only 60% of what my base salary was – and some of that is taxable). It's not easy. I'm very grateful for the good benefits my company provided. By law under COBRA (Consolidated Omnibus Budget Reconciliation Act), after you stop working, you are entitled to continue the health coverage that was provided to you through your employer for a maximum of 18 months. You will have to pay the full premium, but you will not be dropped. There are other provisions that can possibly extend your eligibility. Use the medical social worker at your local medical center to help run interference for you.

An extremely helpful resource is a non-profit organization called the Patient Advocate Foundation. They can provide you with information on everything from how to apply for Social Security Disability to how to appeal insurance decisions. They can help with job discrimination issues and debt crisis, can expedite preauthorization and help you gain access to treatment and medical devices you might need. They also have caseworkers who will do this on your behalf. They exist to serve as a liaison, especially when you might be too ill or overwhelmed to advocate for yourself.

They can be reached at 1 (800) 532-5274 or on the Web at www.patientadvocate.org

Palliative Care and Hospice

I don't know when I might need hospice care, but I hope that my doctor and I will explore it as soon as it seems appropriate. Palliative care, which hospice specializes in, provides treatment of symptoms associated with the final phases of a disease. This generally is offered when the disease itself is no longer being actively treated. It may be that the doctor lets the patient know that all treatment possibilities have been exhausted. Maybe the patient herself decides that she has undergone enough treatment and would prefer to spend her remaining time as comfortable as possible and not debilitated by further treatment.

Hospice care providers are experts in end-of-life care, pain management, and ensuring as high a quality of life as possible at the end stage of a disease. They are specially trained health care and medical personnel who understand the unique issues facing patients and their families at this stage of life. Most hospice care is offered in the home.

Hospice care generally is appropriate when the life expectancy is less than six months. With cancer, and certainly with breast cancer, this isn't always easy to predict. My wish is that as soon as it might be appropriate to use hospice care, I would want to. I've known friends who didn't get the benefit of this level of specialized care or perhaps only had the experts working with them for a few weeks. I've seen what special, tender, and respectful care can be provided through hospice and I would want my family as well as myself to be able to benefit from this special resource. Hospice provides care for the whole family and also helps the family members after the patient dies.

One night in my therapy group for women with advanced breast cancer, we talked about what being referred to hospice meant to us and to those around us. We agreed that often people see it as something you go to at the absolute end. As one of my friends in the group said, "When people hear that you've entered hospice care, they say, 'She's going down!'" This unfortunate perception that seems to be so pervasive keeps many people from using the comprehensive care offered by hospice until the very last days of their lives. Accepting hospice care is not necessarily giving up. It's just acknowledging another phase of your illness and your changing needs.

Interestingly, the friend who shared that observation about how people think of hospice care went home after our meeting and called our local hospice care provider. She had been living with brain metastases and severe headaches and had not been in active treatment for more than six months. She realized after talking it through that the time was right to use hospice. When we met again two weeks later, she shared that she had gotten hospice involved in her care. She was so enthusiastic. Hospice has assessed her pain level and for the first time in over a year, she has adequate pain control. She has a nurse who coordinates all aspects of her care. A counselor had already met with her children. The hospice caseworker had completed a whole needs assessment for her and her family. She's become a hospice "groupie!" She still has good days and bad days. On a good day, she is able to drive and do what she wants to, from attending her son's ballgames to dropping in at her old office. On a bad day, she can call the nurse and receive the appropriate dose of pain medicine to get relief from a severe headache, knowing that a professional is monitoring how she's doing, aware of all aspects of her illness and of the needs of her family. Best of all, she feels that a team of caring people are walking with her through this time in her life, with their primary objective that of being her advocate and ensuring that this is quality time.

She knows that hospice is committed not only to her, but also to her immediate and extended family, now and after she passes. I want that kind of peace of mind and help when the time comes.

End of life issues

If you haven't yet worked with an attorney to draw up a will and make provisions for power of attorney and advance health care directives that make clear what measures you are or are not willing to have at the end of your life, this is the time to do it. Some people think that tending to all of these details is morbid or giving in to the notion of death. I disagree. Doing this kind of planning is the responsible thing to do for yourself and for your family.

I had drawn up a will when my daughter was little. With the progression of my disease, issues that I had decided in the abstract now became concrete and urgent to me. I met with my attorney and revisited many of the provisions of my will, rewriting a good portion of it to reflect changes in my own wishes and changes in the circumstances of my family. It was a great relief to have that resolved. I also reviewed the provisions of my power of attorney arrangements and my advance health care directives, and my doctor has a copy of my document.

Complementary and Alternative Therapies

I've always been a traditional medicine kind of girl, having been raised by a father who was a pharmacist and having been a nurse at one point in my life. When I had my third recurrence, friends and family who had apparently restrained themselves up to this point suddenly began calling, writing and emailing me with every possible alternative therapy they had heard of and the miraculous stories that validated the value of those therapies. I got information on everything from high colonics to Chinese medicine to acupuncture to radical diets. I've thanked each and every one and said that I would review what they sent me – and I have. I've also tried to look for clinical trials that validate the efficacy of these approaches.

I'm still most comfortable with proven medical treatment, but each of us has to pursue what we need to do to feel actively involved in our treatment and to be true to ourselves. I know some people who are strictly going the herbal route. I know someone else who really did high colonics and swore they made her feel better!

While I haven't used herbs or other non-traditional medicine, I have been using massage and Reiki therapy to achieve deep relaxation. The cancer center where I go for treatment has a comprehensive cancer resource facility and they are very committed to the mind/body/spirit connection and supporting care of all aspects of the person who is ill. I have really benefited from these therapies and have learned deep relaxation and breathing techniques. It just makes me feel better, and it's a way of taking care of myself.

There is a complementary and alternative medicine branch of the National Institutes of Health. A lot of research is currently underway to explore the science behind non-traditional approaches that don't follow the conventional Western model of medicine that is the norm here in the US. Go to the nih.gov site and do a search on "complementary and alternative medicine." There is a separate section just on this topic.

If you decide to use any treatments outside of conventional therapy, be sure to let your oncologist know. Sometimes herbs and other things can affect your chemotherapy or other approved treatments.

Being Remembered and Reconciliation

When my granddaughter was born, I realized that I might not be around to see her grow up. None of us has a guarantee anyway, but those of us with advanced breast cancer have the piercing awareness of how important it is to connect now with people we love. I began writing my little granddaughter letters, sharing things that I wanted her to know – about me, about how much I love her, about her family, about life. I wanted to provide a tangible thing for her to go back to, to know about my relationship to her.

After I began writing those letters (which I've done in a journal for her), I began thinking of other people I wanted to let know how much they mean to me. At first, I thought that I would write letters to leave to people. Then I realized that I should still write the letters, but why not give them now? Letting people know how important they are to you can transform and deepen your relationships, and that's a gift to you and to them as well. You can accomplish this through letters or making video or audio tapes. Some people prefer to use the visual arts, including scrap booking.

As I've taken stock of my life and my relationships, there have been a few where I felt that there is unfinished business. I've tried to make peace and finish or reconcile issues where possible. I know that this isn't always possible, but I'm making every reasonable effort. It feels good.

The Ebb and Flow of Decline

Six months ago, I thought that my disease was going to progress rapidly. I felt urgency – almost to the point of desperation -- to tackle things having to do with the end of my life. It was hard work and not easy emotionally, but it was good work.

The course of metastatic breast cancer is not always predictable. This is where you and your doctor need to have a close, open and honest relationship. There are questions that I wonder about that I have chosen not to ask my oncologist yet. I don't want a prediction yet as to how long he thinks I might have to live. I know that I'm suggestible enough that if he said "a year" I'd probably check out a year to the day from that prediction. The time may come when I want him to estimate for me. Other people want to know this estimate so that they are prodded to get their personal affairs in order or to rev up their fighting spirit and say, "No way! I'm going to outlive that estimate by a mile!" Know yourself and what you need to feed your hope.

As so often happens, I got into a deep discussion with another patient in the treatment room about tackling hard issues. He was wrestling with knowing when to stop treatment, being able to decide when the cost of treatment in quality of life and physical terms outweighed the benefit. While he wasn't ready to make that decision yet, he wondered what his doctor's position would be and how hard or easy it would be to discuss that. We talked about the value of speaking with the doctor just about how to begin that conversation so that when the time came to have the real discussion, the door would already be open, even if not yet walked through.

A year ago, I really didn't think that I would be alive now. It goes to show how little I know! I've had to learn to surf the crests and troughs of my physical and emotional state, knowing that the tide of my illness is bearing me onward, but that I can't know all the factors that will influence that tide.

The exercise, discipline, and blessing for me is to live in what Sir William Osler called "day-tight compartments." I'm grateful for today, and I'm going to squeeze every good thing out of it that I can.

Glossary of Medical and Scientific Terms

5-FU – 5 fluorouracil; an anticancer drug that is given intravenously. It is in the class of "antimetabolites" and interferes with the cell's ability to make DNA and RNA, thus making it unable to divide, leading to the death of the cell. It is used in breast cancer and many other kinds of cancer.

Adriamycin – brand name Doxorubicin; an anticancer drug that is given intravenously. In a class of drugs called "anthracyclines," it interferes with the life of the cancer cell at various stages in its metabolism, leading to cell death. It is used in breast cancer and many other kinds of cancer. Sometimes patients call it "red devil" because it is a ruby red solution.

Alimta - generic name pemetrexed; an anticancer drug given intravenously to treat several specific kinds of lung cancer. It is being used experimentally in treating breast cancer that has spread and not responded to other drugs.

Alternative medicine – a treatment or therapy that is used instead of conventional medicine, e.g. using a special diet instead of standard surgery or chemotherapy.

Anemia – a level of red blood cells that is below normal, resulting in fatigue and stress on the body's organs from lack of adequate oxygen. Anemia in breast cancer is usually a side effect of chemotherapy, which can temporarily interfere with the body's ability to produce red blood cells.

Arimidex – generic name anastrozole; an oral anticancer drug used to treat breast cancer in women who have gone through menopause. This is a hormone therapy that blocks the production of estrogen which, in some breast cancer tumors, promotes the growth of the tumor. Specifically, Arimidex is an aromatase inhibitor (see "aromatase inhibitor").

Aromatase inhibitor – a kind of drug that blocks the enzyme aromatase, which normally converts androgens (hormones made in the adrenal glands) into estrogen. Without estrogen, tumors dependent upon it should shrink.

Benadryl – generic name diphenhydramine; an antihistamine; used to prevent or treat allergic reactions.

Biopsy – the removal of a sample of tissue from the body for examination.

Blood count – a common laboratory test using a sample of blood from the patient, which looks at white blood cells, red blood cells, and platelets and can help detect anemia, infections, and potential problems with blood clotting.

Bone scan – a test that detects increased or decreased bone metabolism. A small amount of a radioactive chemical (see "radioactive isotope") is injected into the vein and travels to the bones. A special scanner takes an image of the whole body and a computer generates an image as a picture, which can show abnormal activity. The radioactive chemical tends to concentrate in areas where new bone is being formed. In bone tumors, growth is rapid and therefore shows up on the scan.

Boost treatments - focused radiation usually given upon completion of radiation therapy to deliver a final, intense dose of radiation to the tumor area and hopefully destroy any remaining cancer cells.

Breast prosthesis – an artificial breast form that can be worn after a mastectomy, made from silicone gel, foam, or fiberfill, and usually weighted to appear similar in shape and texture to a natural breast. Some adhere directly to the chest and others are worn in a post-mastectomy bra equipped with a soft pocket into which the prosthesis is placed. Partial prostheses are also available for women who have had a portion of their breast removed.

Breast reconstruction – a plastic surgery procedure to rebuild the contour of the breast, usually including the nipple and areola. There are many options for reconstruction, including those using the patient's own tissue (see "TRAM flap reconstruction") and the use of breast implants (see "reconstruction with implants").

Bronchoscopy - a diagnostic procedure in which a tube using a special camera is inserted through the nose or mouth into the lungs by way of the trachea (windpipe) and bronchial tubes. The procedure provides a view of the airways of the lung and a way to take a tissue sample for examination.

Carboplatin – trade name Paraplatin; an anticancer drug in the class of "alkylating agents" that is given intravenously. Carboplatin affects the cell during its resting phase, directly attacking the DNA. This drug is used in breast cancer and other cancers as well.

Chemotherapy – the use of anticancer drugs to destroy cancer cells; often referred to by patients and medical personnel just as "chemo." There are many different kinds of chemotherapy.

Clinical trial – a drug research study in which people help doctors and scientists determine if newly developed drugs or techniques will be useful and safe in treating a disease (see also "Phase I, Phase II and Phase III clinical trials").

Complementary medicine – a treatment or therapy that is used together with conventional medicine, e.g. massage or meditation.

CT scan – sometimes called a "CAT" scan, computed tomagraphy scan; a special X-ray in which images of the body are obtained from multiple angles and then processed through a computer to show cross sections of body tissues and organs.

Cytoxan – generic name cyclophosphamide; an anticancer drug that is given intravenously. It is an alkylating agent that directly attacks the cancer cell's DNA.

Decadron – generic name dexamethasone; a drug often given in combination with chemotherapy drugs to prevent an allergic reaction.

Dysentery – an illness involving severe diarrhea and intestinal pain resulting from inflammation of the stomach and intestines, caused by ingestion of water or food contaminated with bacteria or a parasitic amoeba.

Epinephrine – an injectable drug used to treat life-threatening allergic reactions. It relaxes the muscles in the airways and constricts the blood vessels, helping to reverse shock.

Estrogen blocker – a broad class of drugs that include various agents that prevent estrogen from binding to the surface of a breast cancer cell. These drugs are used in women who have gone through menopause whose breast cancer tumor cells have special proteins (estrogen receptors) that bind to estrogen, causing the tumor to grow.

Estrogen receptor positive – sometimes informally called "estrogen sensitive"; also known as ER+; a common characteristic of breast cancer cells in which the cell surface has receptor sites for estrogen and in which estrogen enhances the cancer cell's ability to grow and divide.

Femara – generic name letrozole; a form of hormone therapy in the class of aromatase inhibitors (see "aromatase inhibitors").

Frozen section – a technique for examining tissue quickly, e.g. during an operation, in which a pathologist can quick-freeze fresh tissue in order to slice a very thin layer to be examined under a microscope in order to make a preliminary diagnosis.

Gemcitabine – trade name Gemzar; an anticancer drug that is given intravenously. It is in the class of "antimetabolite" and interferes with the cell's ability to make DNA and RNA, thus making it unable to divide, leading to the death of the cell. It is used in breast cancer and many other kinds of cancer.

Gross examination – examination with the naked eye, without the benefit of a microscope or special tools or techniques.

GW572016 – generic name lapatinib, brand name Tykerb; an oral anti-cancer drug still being studied, with some success in patients with advanced breast cancer and in other cancers.

Hemovac – a brand of surgical drain that consists of a round receptacle that collects fluids from the wound through a plastic tube sutured in place. It exerts a small amount of suction to prevent the accumulation of blood and serum in a wound cavity and is very common after a mastectomy or reconstructive surgery.

HER2 – also called erbB2, HER2 stands for human epidermal growth factor receptor 2; HER2 is a gene that helps control how cells grow. If a cell has too many copies of the HER2 gene, it makes too much of a protein that promotes cell growth (called HER2 overexpression). This can lead to cancer and can be a factor in how aggressive the cancer is. About 25% of women with breast cancer have a defect in the HER2 gene.

Herceptin – generic name trastuzumab; this drug is in the class of biologic therapies. It uses a substance taken from living cells and specifically targets the protein on the cells' surface that is made as a result of HER2 overexpression, binding directly with the cancer cells and signaling the body to destroy them. It is sometimes used in combination with chemotherapy drugs. For a fascinating read about the development of this drug, see Robert Bazell's *Her-2: The Making of Herceptin, a Revolutionary Treatment for Breast Cancer.*

Hodgkin's lymphoma – sometimes also called Hodgkin's Disease; a cancer of the lymph tissue found in the lymph nodes, spleen, and bone marrow.

Informed consent – the process by which a patient can understand fully the facts and implications of treatment options and participate in choices about her health care. It is based upon the legal and ethical right the patient has to direct what happens to her body and from the ethical duty of the physician to involve the patient in her health care.

Infusion pump – an electronically powered, compact, portable pump used to deliver intravenous chemotherapy into the bloodstream in small, controlled doses over long periods of time.

Inner quadrant – Dividing the breast into imaginary quarters like pie slices, inner quadrant tumors occur in the upper or lower sections close to the breastbone (as opposed to the armpit). Tumor distribution in breast cancer is roughly 50% in the upper outer quadrant, 20% in the central portion near the nipple, 10 % in the lower outer quadrant, 10% in the upper inner quadrant, and 10% in the lower inner quadrant.

Invasive breast cancer – also called "infiltrating," these breast cancers have broken through the breast's milk ducts or lobules and have started to spread to surrounding breast tissue. Most breast cancers are detected when they have already reached this stage.

IV – Intravenous; a method of administering medication directly into the vein.

Lesion – a non-specific term that refers to abnormal tissue in the body.

Lobular breast cancer – a type of breast cancer that arises in the lobes of the breast where milk is manufactured. This type of breast cancer accounts for about 10% of all breast cancers. It often appears as a thickening in the breast tissue rather than a well-defined lump. The most common form of breast cancer is ductal (accounting for about 80%), which arises in the microscopic tubes that transport the milk to the nipple.

Lumpectomy – surgery to remove only the cancerous lump and a small amount of surrounding tissue, thus conserving breast tissue.

Lymph node – part of the body's lymphatic system, which also includes lymph vessels and some organs (e.g. the spleen). Lymph fluid circulates in this system, carrying waste products away from the cells' fluids and returning them to the bloodstream to be eliminated from the body. Lymph nodes filter out and trap bacteria, viruses, cancer cells, and other unwanted substances.

Malignant – in medical terms, harmful; most often used to mean cancerous.

Margins – the edges of tissue that has been removed; "Clean" or "clear" margins means that there is no microscopic evidence of any cancerous cells on the outermost edges of the tissue specimen. "Dirty" or "Positive" margins means that cancer cells were still evident and further surgery may be necessary to cut the area more widely to try to ensure that all of the cancer cells have been removed from that area.

Mastectomy – surgical removal of the entire breast (see "modified radical mastectomy" and "simple mastectomy").

Metastasis/metastatic disease – the spread of cancer to a new part of the body, which occurs usually through the blood or lymph system. Breast cancer most commonly spreads to the bones, liver, or lungs and sometimes to the brain.

Methotrexate – brand name Trexall; an anticancer drug that is given intravenously. It is in the class of "antimetabolites" and interferes with the cell's ability to make DNA, thus making it unable to divide, leading to the death of the cell. It is used in breast cancer and many other kinds of cancer. It also is used for other medical purposes, including treating rheumatoid arthritis.

Modified radical mastectomy – a surgical procedure that removes the entire breast and the lymph nodes in the adjacent armpit. Prior to the 1980's, a more extensive surgery was routinely done, using the techniques developed by the pioneering surgeon, William Halsted, in the late 1800's. For nearly 100 years, the main treatment for breast cancer was a "Halsted radical mastectomy," which removed the breast, lymph nodes, and also the underlying chest muscle. Research has shown that unless the breast cancer has spread to the chest muscle, necessitating that it be removed, patients do equally well with the modified version of the surgery that spares the chest muscle and causes less disfigurement and loss of function in the arm.

MRI – magnetic resonance imaging; a diagnostic method that uses radiofrequency waves and a strong magnetic field (instead of x-rays) to create detailed images of internal organs and tissue.

Multidisciplinary team conference – a consultation between all the members of the patient's health care team (e.g. surgeon, oncologist, radiation oncologist, pathologist, oncology nurse, social worker, etc.) to review the patient's current status and treatment options and to reach consensus on recommendations for the patient. Ideally, the conference ultimately invites the patient and/or caregiver to speak with the team, too, after they have consulted.

Needle biopsy – sometimes called "fine needle biopsy," "fine needle aspiration" or "FNA"; This technique uses a thin needle through the skin into the breast tissue to extract either fluid or cells from a questionable area to examine under a microscope. Other types of biopsies can also be performed with larger sized needles that can take a core of tissue for examination, some of which are done with the use of imaging equipment.

Neupogen – generic name filgrastim; a drug given by injection that stimulates the bone marrow to produce white blood cells. It is used when a patient's white blood cell count dips to potentially dangerous levels, to reduce the chances of infection. A longer lasting drug in this same class called Neulasta is also sometimes used. Keeping the white blood cell count closer to normal can enable the patient to take the course of chemotherapy at the full dose without interruption.

Neutropenia – low white blood cell count, specifically of white blood cells called neutrophils, which are important in fighting off infections. It is a frequent side effect of cancer chemotherapy.

Nodule – a small, solid collection of tissue that can be felt.

Oncologist – a physician with special training who studies, diagnoses, and treats cancer. This specialty can be further divided into medical oncology, surgical oncology, and radiation oncology.

Open biopsy – a surgical procedure that removes part or all of the questionable tissue for examination and diagnosis.

Pathology – the branch of medical science that deals with the nature, causes, and development of diseases at a cellular level. The pathologist makes the diagnosis of disease based upon tissues and fluids removed from the body.

Pathology report - the written report of the pathologist of his/her findings from examination of the specimen with the naked eye, under the microscope, and through various tests. This report helps guide the oncologist in treatment decisions.

Permanent breast implant – a breast form filled either with silicone or saline solution that, in the case of breast reconstruction, is surgically placed under the chest muscle, in the pocket created through tissue expansion. Some surgeons prefer to use a combination expander/implant rather than two separate devices (see also "tissue expander").

PET scan – Positron Emission Tomography; a diagnostic examination that detects the emission of positrons, specific atomic particles given off from an intravenous solution administered to the patient. A glucose compound "tagged" with a radioactive substance is given. Since tumors grow at a faster rate than normal, healthy tissue, they take up the radioactive glucose more readily and therefore give off more positrons. When the body is scanned, "hot spots" that are likely tumor growth are then visible. PET scans are also used to evaluate other medical conditions.

Pharmacokinetics – the study of what the body does with a drug, e.g. how it is metabolized and excreted and what its active levels in the blood are at various times after it is administered to the patient.

Phase I clinical trial – first time use of a drug in a small group of humans to test its safety, determine a safe dose range, and identify side effects.

Phase II clinical trial – expanded use of an experimental drug or treatment to a larger group of people than a Phase I trial to test its effectiveness and to evaluate further its safety.

Phase III clinical trial – the administration of an experimental drug or treatment to a large group of people to confirm Phase II findings about the drug's effectiveness, to compare its effectiveness with existing approved and commonly used treatments, to continue to track side effects, and to collect information that will allow the drug to be used safely.

Platelets – also called "thrombocytes"; specialized fragments of large bone marrow cells with sticky surfaces that make them clump together, which is an essential part of forming a blood clot to stop bleeding. Some cancer drugs reduce the number of platelets.

Port-a-cath – a brand name that has become a generic term for a special intravenous device surgically implanted in the subclavian vein, a large vein under the collarbone; sometimes also just called a "port." This device provides access for chemotherapy through a quarter-sized disc under the skin, into which the IV needle is insert-ed. Advantages include not having to find a vein in the arm every time for treatments and virtual elimination of the danger of caustic chemotherapy drugs leaking into surrounding tissues, which can happen if an IV in the arm slips out of position and the medicine infiltrates the area outside of the vein. Even patients with "good veins" in their arms may experience hardening or scarring in the veins from chemotherapy, so ports are widely used. Blood samples can also be drawn for most lab tests via the Port-a-cath.

Pre-op – before a surgical operation.

Preventive or prophylactic mastectomy – elective surgical removal of one or both breasts to prevent or reduce the risk of breast cancer in women at high risk for the disease.

Radiation recall – a skin reaction associated with certain chemotherapy drugs administered after a patient has received radiation therapy, characterized by symptoms replicating a burn, with sunburn-like redness, pain, swelling, tenderness and sometimes even peeling skin and wet sores, and which occurs in the area where a patient had received radiation therapy in the past.

Radiation simulation – the planning portion of radiation therapy in which every aspect of the patient's treatment is rehearsed as closely as possible to what the actual treatment will entail. This includes positioning the patient, marking the patient, providing custom-made blocks to shield healthy tissue and cushions to help keep the patient in an exact place on the treatment table, and CT scans or x-rays to enable the radiation oncologist and his/her team to design the treatment in minute and specific detail.

Radiation therapy – also called "radiotherapy," "irradiation" and "x-ray therapy"; the treatment of disease using very targeted high energy waves or streams of atomic particles to penetrate the diseased area to kill the affected cells or keep them from growing.

Radioactive isotope – sometimes also called "radioactive tracer"; a specially created form of a chemical element that has an extra neutron. Because it is unstable and seeks to go back to its natural form, it emits low levels of atomic radiation that can be scanned or otherwise detected and interpreted as an image.

Reconstruction with implants – a method of breast reconstruction in which the plastic surgeon creates a pocket under the chest muscle (pectoral muscle) that is expanded over time and eventually receives a permanent breast form filled with saline solution or silicone to create a breast mound, simulating the contour of a natural breast. The surgeon can also create a nipple and areola, using the patient's own tissue or cartilage and tattooing the area to a natural shade.

Recurrence – the return and reappearance of cancer after primary treatment has been completed.

Regional recurrence – the return of breast cancer to the general vicinity of the original tumor, including the chest wall and nearby lymph nodes, but not to other distant organs (e.g. bones, liver, lungs).

Reiki – a Japanese technique for stress reduction and deep relaxation that uses light, sustained touch.

Remission – sometimes charactized as complete or partial; complete remission is when there is no clinical evidence by examination or any other diagnostic test that any cancer is present in the body. Partial remission is when the tumor or tumors have shrunk but are still present.

Saline solution – salt in sterile water, usually in a concentration that replicates that of the human body (0.9%).

Simple mastectomy – removal of the entire breast but not any lymph nodes. Usually done for preventive purposes.

Sternum – the breastbone.

Steroid – Steroids used in cancer care are in the same family as those naturally produced by the adrenal glands. They are given to help prevent allergic reactions to some chemotherapy drugs or to transfusions, to help prevent nausea and vomiting, and to reduce inflammation.

Systemic – affecting the whole body; systemic chemotherapy affects cancer cells that may be present anywhere in the body, not just at the site of the tumor.

Tamoxifen – brand name "Nolvadex"; an oral hormone therapy that blocks the effects of estrogen. Once given routinely to postmenopausal women with estrogen receptor positive tumors, it is being replaced largely by the aromatase inhibitors, like Arimidex and Femara.

Taxol – generic name paclitaxel; an anticancer drug in the plant alkaloid family, it is a "taxane," derived from the Pacific yew tree. It is given intravenously and acts by affecting the microtubule structure within cancer cells, interfering with cell division and thus causing cell death. It is used in breast cancer and other cancers.

Taxotere – generic name docetaxel; a synthetic anticancer drug in the plant alkaloid family, it is a taxane. It is given intravenously and acts by affecting the microtubule structure within cancer cells, interfering with cell division and thus causing cell death. It is used in breast cancer and other cancers.

Thoracic – pertaining to the thorax (the chest).

Tissue expander – a silicone balloon that is placed under skin or muscle and expanded with saline solution over time, causing the skin to stretch and grow so that reconstructive surgery can be performed.

TRAM flap reconstruction – TRAM stands for transverse rectus abdominis muscle; a method of breast reconstruction surgery that uses the patient's own tissue, in which an oval portion of skin, fat and abdominal muscle is moved from the lower abdomen up under the tissue and onto the chest to create a natural looking breast.

Tumor – an abnormal growth of tissue that forms a mass; it may or may not be cancerous.

Ultrasound – a diagnostic technique that uses sound waves beyond human hearing and their echoes to create an image. Ultrasound can help determine if a lump is solid or filled with fluid.

Vasculitis – inflammation of the blood vessels.

Versed – a sedative often used before surgery to relax the patient and decrease memory of the events around the time of surgery.

White count/white blood cell count – a blood test to determine the level of white blood cells and the relative number of the different kinds of white blood cells. This test helps detect infections or increased risk of infections during chemotherapy.

Xeloda – generic name capecitabine; an oral anticancer drug in the family of anti-metabolites. It is metabolized into 5-FU and interferes with the cell's ability to make DNA and RNA, thus making it unable to divide, leading to the death of the cell. It is used in breast cancer and other kinds of cancer.

Zofran – generic name odansetron; an anti-emetic drug used to control nausea and vomiting. The mechanism of Zofran, Kytril, and other newer anti-emetics like Emend and Aloxi is very specific and different than other antinausea drugs like Phenergan or Torecan and provides an invaluable addition to the ways to prevent or control nausea and vomiting. Drugs like Zofran attach to specific cell receptor sites and help prevent the cascade of biochemical events that cause severe nausea and vomiting.

Bibliography

Poems of Rumi that appear in *Slapped Awake* are referenced in two ways in this bibliography section. First, there is a listing of titles of books of the translator Coleman Barks, noting in which book the full text of each poem appears. Second, there is a listing by *Slapped Awake* chapter, arranged in numerical order, cross-referencing the section of each poem appearing in the chapters' epigraphs back to Barks's books.

Books by Coleman Barks

Slapped Awake chapter number in which the quote appears is in parentheses.

Rumi, Jalaluddin; Coleman Barks, translator, *Birdsong,* Maypop Books, Athens, GA Copyright 1993
    "Birds make great sky-circles…" pg. 13 (chapter 1)
    "We search this world…" pg. 17 (chapter 3)

Rumi, Jalaluddin; Coleman Barks, translator, *The Essential Rumi*; HarperCollins Publishers, Harper San Francisco, copyright 1995

      "The Guest House," pg. 109

      "Late by myself…" pg. 12 (chapter 2)

      "A night full of talking…" pg. 50 (chapter 5)

      "It's a drum and arms waving…" pg. 95 (chapter 6)

      "The morning wind spreads…" pg. 267 (chapter 7)

      "You are so weak. Give up to grace." pg. 70 (chapter 8)

      "Last year, I gazed at the fire…" pg. 7 (chapter 10)

      "The light changes…" pg. 53 (chapter 11)

      "Today, like every other day…" pg. 36 (chapter 14)

      "Dance, when you're broken open." pg. 281 (chapter 16)

Rumi, Jalaluddin; Coleman Barks, translator; *The Soul of Rumi*; HarperCollins Publishers, Harper San Francisco, copyright 2001

      "Everyone chooses a suffering…" pg. 25 (chapter 4)

      "Longing is the core of mystery…" pg. 96 (chapter 9)

      "Be ground. Be crumbled…" pg. 21 (chapter 12)

      "The center leads to love." pg. 174 (chapter 13)

      "I placed one foot on the wide plain…" pg. 96 (chapter 15),

Rumi, Jalaluddin; Coleman Barks, translator; *Unseen Rain*; Threshold Books, Putney, VT, copyright 1986

      "Life is ending? God gives another." pg. 9 (chapter 17),

Slapped Awake Chapter Epigraphs

Rumi poetry sources are cross-referenced by epigraphs to chapters in *Slapped Awake*.

Chapter 1: "Birds make great sky-circles..."
Rumi, Jalaluddin; Coleman Barks, translator, *Birdsong*, Maypop Books, Athens, GA Copyright 1993, pg. 13

Chapter 2: "Late, by myself..."
Rumi, Jalaluddin; Coleman Barks, translator, *The Essential Rumi*; HarperCollins Publishers, Harper San Francisco, copyright 1995, pg. 12

Chapter 3: "We search this world..."
Rumi, Jalaluddin; Coleman Barks, translator, *Birdsong*, Maypop Books, Athens, GA Copyright 1993, pg 17

Chapter 4: "Everyone chooses a suffering..."
Rumi, Jalaluddin; Coleman Barks, translator; *The Soul of Rumi*; HarperCollins Publishers, Harper San Francisco, copyright 2001, pg. 25 (excerpted from "Choose a Suffering")

Chapter 5: "A night full of talking..."
Rumi, Jalaluddin; Coleman Barks, translator, *The Essential Rumi*; HarperCollins Publishers, Harper San Francisco, copyright 1995, pg. 50

Chapter 6: "It's a drum and arms waving..."
Rumi, Jalaluddin; Coleman Barks, translator, *The Essential Rumi*; HarperCollins Publishers, Harper San Francisco, copyright 1995, pg. 95 (excerpted from "Bonfire at Midnight")

Chapter 7: "The morning wind spreads its fresh smell..."
Rumi, Jalaluddin; Coleman Barks, translator, *The Essential Rumi*; HarperCollins Publishers, Harper San Francisco, copyright 1995, pg. 267

Chapter 8:   "You are so weak. Give up to grace."
Rumi, Jalaluddin; Coleman Barks, translator, *The Essential Rumi*; HarperCollins Publishers, Harper San Francisco, copyright 1995, pg. 70 (excerpted from "Bismallah")

Chapter 9:   "Longing is the core of mystery…"
Rumi, Jalaluddin; Coleman Barks, translator; *The Soul of Rumi*; HarperCollins Publishers, Harper San Francisco, copyright 2001, pg. 96

Chapter 10:   "Last year, I gazed at the fire…"
Rumi, Jalaluddin; Coleman Barks, translator, *The Essential Rumi*; HarperCollins Publishers, Harper San Francisco, copyright 1995, pg. 7 (excerpted from "Burnt Kabob")

Chapter 11:   "The light changes…"
Rumi, Jalaluddin; Coleman Barks, translator, *The Essential Rumi*; HarperCollins Publishers, Harper San Francisco, copyright 1995, pg. 53

Chapter 12:   "Be ground. Be crumbled…"
Rumi, Jalaluddin; Coleman Barks, Translator; *The Soul of Rumi*; HarperCollins Publishers, Harper San Francisco, copyright 2001, pg. 21 (excerpted from "A Necessary Autumn Inside Each")

Chapter 13:   "The center leads to love."
Rumi, Jalaluddin; Coleman Barks, Translator; *The Soul of Rumi*; HarperCollins Publishers, Harper San Francisco, copyright 2001, pg. 174

Chapter 14:   "Today, like every other day…"
Rumi, Jalaluddin; Coleman Barks, translator, *The Essential Rumi*;

HarperCollins Publishers, Harper San Francisco, copyright 1995, pg. 36

Chapter 15: "I placed one foot on the wide plain..."
Rumi, Jalaluddin; Coleman Barks, Translator; *The Soul of Rumi*; HarperCollins Publishers, Harper San Francisco, copyright 2001, pg. 96

Chapter 16: "Dance, when you're broken open."
Rumi, Jalaluddin; Coleman Barks, translator, *The Essential Rumi*; HarperCollins Publishers, Harper San Francisco, copyright 1995, pg. 281

Chapter 17: "Life is ending? God gives another."
Rumi, Jalaludding; Coleman Barks, translator; *Unseen Rain*; Threshold Books, Putney, VT, copyright 1986, pg. 9

For More Information

National Cancer Institute

(800) 4-CANCER www.cancer.gov

The National Institutes for Health's arm for addressing cancer in the U.S., the National Cancer Institute conducts and supports research, training, health information, and other programs addressing the cause, diagnosis, prevention, and treatment of cancer, rehabilitation from cancer, and the continuing care of cancer patients and the families of cancer patients. They have up-to-date information on specific cancer diagnoses and treatments available, including clinical trials.

Y-ME National Breast Cancer Organization, Inc.

(800) 221-2141 (24/7 hotline) www.y-me.org

The mission of Y-ME is to ensure, through information, empowerment and peer support, that no one faces breast cancer alone. Y-ME helps women with breast cancer and their families through a hotline for information and peer support, support groups, education, and information. Peer support and information on the hotline is available in English and Spanish, and translation is available in over 150 languages.

Chemocare
www.chemocare.com
Visit this site for information on all types of cancer treatment, including tips for dealing with side effects. This web resource is sponsored by Olympic champion figure skater Scott Hamilton, who has been treated for testicular cancer.

National Center for Complementary and Alternative Medicine
www.nccam.nih.gov
The National Institute for Health's own center is helpful for the latest news and research, including clinical trials, available for complementary therapies.

Young Survival Coalition
www.youngsurvival.org
Services focus on the issues facing women under 40 who are diagnosed with breast cancer.

Sisters Network, Inc.
www.sistersnetworkinc.org
This organization's aim is to increase national and local attention to the impact of breast cancer in the African-American community.

Patient Advocate Foundation
(800) 532-5274 www.patientadvocate.org
This organization offers legal counseling, case management, referrals, and advocacy on behalf of cancer patients and survivors on issues including insurance and managed care, financial issues, job discrimination, and disability.

Coleman Barks and Rumi

www.colemanbarks.com

The site for writer and translator Coleman Barks, this resource tells about his most recent work and has many links for more information about the poet Rumi.

The Baha'i Faith

(800) 22-UNITE   www.bahai.us

The official US website for the Baha'i Faith provides information on the core beliefs and history of the faith, news, areas of social action, how to access publications, links to some of the Baha'i scriptures, and how to get more information on Baha'is in the United States. For an overview of the international Baha'i community and links to websites of Baha'i communities in other countries, see www.bahai.org

Deborah Lang Hampton is a writer and poet whose varied career has included work as a philanthropy professional, editor of a national children's magazine, medical and scientific writer and editor, musician, and registered nurse. She lives in Chattanooga, Tennessee, with her husband and their children and grandchildren.

www.slappedawake.com
deborahhampton@slappedawake.com

Printed in the United States
72900LV00001B/1-135